ABOUT CANADA
HEALTH AND ILLNESS

ABOUT CANADA
HEALTH AND ILLNESS

Dennis Raphael

About Canada Series

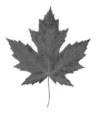

Fernwood Publishing • Halifax & Winnipeg

Editing: Robert Clarke
Cover design: John van der Woude
Text design: Brenda Conroy
Printed and bound in Canada by Hignell Printing

Mixed Sources
Product group from well-managed forests and other controlled sources
www.fsc.org Cert no. SW-COC-003438
© 1996 Forest Stewardship Council
FSC

Published in Canada by Fernwood Publishing
32 Oceanvista Lane, Black Point, Nova Scotia, B0J 1B0
and 748 Broadway Avenue, Winnipeg, MB R3G 0X3
www.fernwoodpublishing.ca

Fernwood Publishing Company Limited gratefully acknowledges the financial support of the Government of Canada through the Canada Book Fund, the Canada Council for the Arts, the Nova Scotia Department of Tourism and Culture and the Province of Manitoba, through the Book Publishing Tax Credit, for our publishing program.

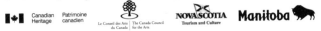

Canadian Heritage Patrimoine canadien   Le Conseil des Arts du Canada | The Canada Council for the Arts   NOVA SCOTIA Tourism and Culture   Manitoba

Library and Archives Canada Cataloguing in Publication

Raphael, Dennis
About Canada : health and illness / Dennis Raphael.

(About Canada)
Includes bibliographical references.
ISBN 978-1-55266-375-2 (pbk.).--ISBN 978-1-55266-388-2 (bound)

1. Public health--Social aspects--Canada. 2. Public health--Economic aspects--Canada. 3. Medical policy—Social aspects--Canada. 4. Social medicine--Canada. I. Title. II. Series: About Canada series

RA418.3.C3R36 2010   362.10971   C2010-902719-1

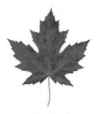

CONTENTS

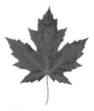

1. WHO STAYS HEALTHY? WHO GETS SICK?

A health care system — even the best health care system in the world — will be only one of the ingredients that determine whether your life will be long or short, healthy or sick, full of fulfillment, or empty with despair. — The Hon. Roy Romanow, 2009

"It's not as if we won't die. We all die," Nancy Krieger of Harvard University's School of Public Health reminds us. "The question is: At what age? With what degree of suffering? With what degree of preventable illness?"[1]

Staying healthy by avoiding disease and early death is undoubtedly one of the greatest concerns in the lives of all Canadians. But how do we go about making that happen? What do we know about keeping Canadians alive and well for as long as possible?

When it comes to issues of health and physical well-being, Canadians tend to pay a lot of attention to medical treatment — especially access to doctors and hospitals — and to making "healthy lifestyle choices." Newspapers and other media are filled with urgent information about hospital budgets, the supply of doctors, or what to eat and how to exercise. But decades of research and hundreds of studies in Canada and elsewhere tell a different story: the primary factors that shape the health and well-being of Canadians — the factors that will give us longer, better lives — are to be found *not* in those much-discussed areas, but rather in the actual living conditions that Canadians experience on a daily basis.

Those conditions include factors such as income and wealth, whether or not we are employed — and, if so, the working conditions we experience — the health services and social services we receive, and our ability to obtain high-quality education, food, and housing, among others. Contrary to the assumption that we have personal control over these factors, in most cases these living conditions are — for better or worse — *imposed* upon us in the normal course of everyday life.

The World Health Organization applies the term "social determinants of health" to these health-influencing factors. It is a term that has come into more and more use in the last couple of decades; a term that, in a nutshell, refers to the social and economic factors that shape the health and incidence of illness among individuals and groups of individuals.[2] The Canadian Senate has also recognized the importance of the social determinants of health. In 2006 it authorized the Standing Senate Committee on Social Affairs, Science and Technology and its Population Health subcommittee to:

> Examine and report on the impact of the multiple factors and conditions that contribute to the health of Canada's population — known collectively as the social determinants of health — including the effects of these determinants on the disparities and inequities in health outcomes that continue to be experienced by identifiable groups or categories of people within the Canadian population.[3]

In addition, the quality of these health-shaping living conditions is strongly determined by the economic system that we live in, and the decisions made by governments and policy-makers. The term "economic system" refers to the means by which economic resources are created and distributed. In Canada the distribution of resources is largely determined by the operation of a market economy, and in order to survive the great majority of individuals in our society must participate in that economy.

The term "government" refers to the elected legislatures in Ottawa, the provinces, and cities that pass laws and regulations that give direction and form to public policy. These public policies can attempt to reduce, ignore, or even magnify the social and health inequalities created by the unmanaged operation of the market economy. The term "policy-maker" refers to government advisors and civil servants who advise elected members of these governments on what public policies to create and implement.

While all wealthy industrialized nations operate within market economies, governments at the municipal, provincial/territorial, and federal levels create and enact policies, laws, and regulations that influence how much income Canadians receive through employment, family benefits, or social assistance. These same structures influence the quality and availability of affordable housing, the health and social services and recreational opportunities available, and even what happens when Canadians lose their jobs during economic downturns such as the one that Canada began experiencing in 2008.

Governments also determine whether our children have access to affordable and high-quality child care and better-quality schools, the working conditions that we experience, and whether as seniors we receive levels of public pensions that allow us to live in dignity. These areas of public policy-making have always been known to influence the quality of life, but they are now also being recognized as primary influences upon our health — as being among those social determinants of health.

The interaction of the economic system with governmental public policy determines in large part the social determinants of health that have such a great impact on the quality of Canadians' lives and well-being. In Canada the strongest supporters of Canada's market economy — the business sector — constantly lobby for policies favoured by owners and managers as opposed to the interests of workers. The business sector also lobbies governments to provide fewer economic supports and services to citizens. The balance between these interests is an important part of the social determinants of health story.

These social determinants are crucial factors in the health and well-being of Canadians. If we can understand how and why they work — and how our services and institutions can be strengthened and our resources more equitably distributed — we will also be able to understand and act to improve the factors that allow us to live longer and healthier lives.

Historical Perspectives on Health and Illness

A concern with what we now call the social determinants of health is nothing new. In the 4th century B.C. the Greek philosopher Plato considered how living conditions — particularly inequality — were shaping health. In *The Laws*, he commented:

> The form of law which I should propose as the natural sequel would be as follows: In a state which is desirous of

---

Friedrich Engels on the Determinants of Workers' Health in England

"All conceivable evils are heaped upon the poor.... They are given damp dwellings, cellar dens that are not waterproof from below or garrets that leak from above.... They are supplied bad, tattered, or rotten clothing, adulterated and indigestible food. They are exposed to the most exciting changes of mental condition, the most violent vibrations between hope and fear.... They are deprived of all enjoyments except sexual indulgence and drunkenness and are worked every day to the point of complete exhaustion of their mental and physical energies."

Source: Friedrich Engels, *The Condition of the Working Class in England* (New York: Penguin Classics, 1987 [1845]), p. 129.

being saved from the greatest of all plagues — not faction, but rather distraction; there should exist among the citizens neither extreme poverty, nor, again, excess of wealth, for both are productive of both these evils.

During the mid-nineteenth century, the German political economist Friedrich Engels showed how the adverse living situations of working-class people in England led to the infections and diseases associated with disease and early death. In his book *The Condition of the Working Class in England* Engels was prescient in his conclusions. Like modern-day health researchers he recognized that unhealthy living conditions, day-to-day stress, and the adoption of health-threatening coping behaviours were the primary causes of disease and early death.

Around the same time, medical doctor Rudolph Virchow was arguing that health-threatening living conditions were rooted in public policy-making. He thereby identified the role that politics played in promoting health and preventing disease. His 1845 *Report*

Rudolf Virchow and the Social Determinants of Health

German physician Rudolf Virchow's (1821–1902) medical discoveries are so extensive that he is known as the "Father of Modern Pathology." But he was also a trailblazer in identifying how societal policies shape health. Virchow stated, "Disease is not something personal and special, but only a manifestation of life under modified (pathological) conditions." Arguing that "medicine is a social science and politics is nothing else but medicine on a large scale," Virchow drew a direct link between social conditions and health: "If medicine is to fulfil her great task, then she must enter the political and social life. Do we not always find the diseases of the populace traceable to defects in society?"

Source: R. Virchow, *Collected Essays on Public Health and Epidemiology* (Cambridge: Science History Publications 1985 [1848]).

on the Typhus Epidemic in Upper Silesia — a Polish province of Prussia — concluded that the lack of democracy, feudal practices, and unfair tax policies led to the inhabitants' poor living conditions, inadequate diet, and problems of hygiene; and he argued that these conditions fuelled the typhus epidemic. Since then, public health authorities' concern with societal conditions and how they shape health and cause illness has never disappeared, but it has always competed with biomedical — and more recently, "healthy lifestyles" — approaches to disease prevention.

A resurgence of interest in the societal causes of health and illness can be traced to the 1980 *Black Report* and the 1987 volume *The Health Divide.*[4] These U.K. reports described how — despite universal access to health care — the lowest occupational-status Britons had the greatest likelihood of suffering from a wide range of diseases and of dying prematurely from illness or injury at every stage of the life cycle. These health differences occurred in a step-by-step progression. Professionals had the best health; skilled workers had moderate health; and manual labourers experienced the worst health. The authors concluded that these inequalities in health were primarily due to differences in concrete living conditions, and not to differences in health attitudes or behaviours. In 1998 another U.K. government inquiry into health inequalities came to similar conclusions about the importance of living conditions as the primary determinants of health.[5]

Canadian Perspectives

Over the years Canadian studies also made contributions to the international understanding of how living conditions and public policies determine health. In 1974 a federal government report, *A New Perspective on the Health of Canadians*, was one of the first modern statements to specify that the environment — broadly defined — played an important role in shaping health. Another Canadian government document, *Achieving Health for All: A Framework for Health*

Promotion, argued in 1986 that health could be improved through the implementation of public policies that would provide Canadians with more secure living conditions.[6]

Canadian Public Health Association (CPHA) documents tell a similar story. The 1996 *Action Statement for Health Promotion in Canada* identified the advocating of new public policies as the single best strategy to improve the health of Canadians. CPHA said that the government should give it priority to reduce the income gap between the rich and poor and to helping communities overcome unhealthy living conditions. In 2000 the association also endorsed an action plan that recognized poverty as a profound threat to health and called for its reduction. These and other CPHA reports drew attention to the harmful health effects of unemployment, income insecurity, homelessness, and insecure economic conditions.[7]

For its part, the Canadian Senate has produced five reports emphasizing the importance of the social determinants of health and of working to improve the prevailing conditions.

The recently concluded work of the World Health Organization's Commission on Social Determinants of Health saw significant Canadian involvement. Canadian government agencies provided funding to the Commission, and Monique Bégin, the former federal minister of Health and Welfare, and Stephen Lewis, the former Canadian ambassador to the United Nations, served as commissioners.[8] Canadian researchers were actively involved with several of the knowledge networks. The final report of the Commission and the reports of its various knowledge hubs have the potential to increase debate on how Canada should address the social determinants of health.

The Social Determinants of Health: How Important Are They?

The nature and extent of health inequalities — which are primarily a result of differences in living conditions — provide good indicators of the role that the social determinants of health play in everyday life and well-being.

The term "health inequalities" refers to the measurable differences in health outcomes that exist among Canadians of differing incomes, genders, or races or other characteristics. There are two main approaches to measuring these inequalities. The first method focuses on measures associated with death (or mortality). These indicators include life expectancy, the number of years of life lost prior to a specific age, say seventy-five years, infant mortality rates, and death rates from various diseases or injuries. The second approach focuses on the presence of disease and injuries, or morbidity (sickness), and includes measures such as low birth-weight rates and the incidence (new cases) and prevalence (total cases) of diseases and injuries. The approaches usually include evidence of poor health outcomes based on objective or subjective reports of health status as indicated by Canadians.

Inequalities in Life Expectancy and Death Rates or Mortality

Not surprisingly, Canadians do not all live to the same age. Even though our average life expectancy is about eighty years, a considerable variation exists. How long Canadians live depends in large part on their incomes. One way of studying this factor is to look at life expectancy in relation to the average income of a neighbourhood. Men living in the poorest 20 percent of urban neighbourhoods in Canada live almost four and a half years less than do those in the wealthiest 20 percent of neighbourhoods. The corresponding figure for women is almost two years less.

Life expectancy also shows a "social gradient": Canadians from the poorest to the wealthiest neighbourhoods have differing average life expectancies. Infant mortality rates follow roughly the same patterns. Infant mortality is said to be an especially sensitive indicator of societal health, and the rates in the poorest urban neighbourhoods are 40 percent higher (7.1/1000) than in the wealthiest neighbourhoods (5/1000). [9]

Death rates among Canadians from diabetes are also strongly

Figure 1-1. Life Expectancy of Males and Females by Income Quintile of Neighbourhood, Urban Canada, 2001

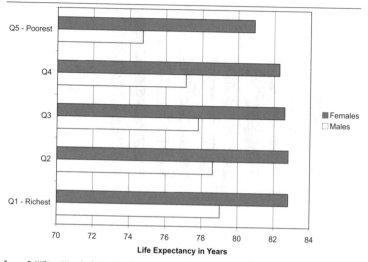

Source: R. Wilkins, "Mortality by Neighbourhood Income in Urban Canada from 1971 to 2001," Statistics Canada, Health Analysis and Measurement Group (HAMG). HAMG Seminar and special compilations, 2007

related to the average income of urban neighbourhoods. In 1971 the death rates from diabetes in wealthy and poor neighbourhoods showed hardly any differences. The situation improved until the mid-1980s, when death rates showed an increase, which was especially the case in lower-income communities. Indeed, there seemed to be a growing epidemic of death from diabetes among lower-income Canadians — and it has since continued to intensify. (The change is not due to the aging of the population because figures have been corrected for increases in age.)

Inequalities in Sickness and Injuries

The incidence of low birth weight across Canada is also a function of average neighbourhood income: rates are 40 percent higher in the poorest neighbourhoods (7/100) as compared to the wealthiest

Figure 1-2. Greater Risk of Injury among Lower Socioeconomic Children, Ontario 1996

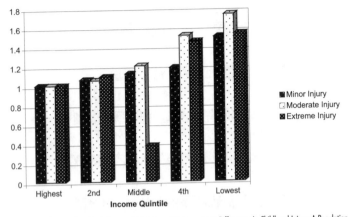

Data adapted from T. Faelker, W. Pickett, and R.J. Brison, "Socioeconomic Differences In Childhood Injury: A Population Based Epidemiologic Study in Ontario, Canada," *Injury Prevention* 6: 203–208, Table 4, p. 206, 2000.

neighbourhoods (4.9/100).[10] A low birth-weight rate is an important indicator of health because it is associated with a wide range of health problems across the lifespan. The same patterns hold for childhood injury.[11] For minor, moderate, and extreme types of injuries, children living in the poorest neighbourhoods had injury rates that were 67 percent higher than that of children living in the wealthiest neighbourhoods.

Getting to the Roots of the Issue: Genetics, Risk Factors, and Risk Conditions

Given that diseases undermine the workings of our bodies, it has been argued that unlocking the human genome will lead to the end of illness as we know it. There is little evidence to support this idea. Very few diseases are caused by the operation of a single or even multiple genes — Huntington's chorea comes to mind — and even when such genes are found they usually provide only a small clue as to whether an individual will get a disease. Discoveries related to the human genome certainly will not influence the health of Canadians in general, especially in regards to the main killers of cancers, heart disease, and respiratory disease.[12]

A similar situation exists in regard to risk factors or what has come to be known as "healthy lifestyle choices." Canadians are now well aware of what U.K. sociologist Sarah Nettleton calls the "holy trinity of risk": unhealthy diet, lack of physical activity, and tobacco use. Indeed, a national survey found that Canadians have over-whelmingly learned and internalized these messages.[13] Disturbingly, this same study found that Canadians have virtually no knowledge of how their health is profoundly shaped by the living conditions, including the social determinants of health that in turn shape their experience.

There is no doubt that, all things being equal, it is better for your health to eat a nutritious diet, be physically active, and avoid tobacco and excessive alcohol use. But the pervasive and narrow focus on "risk factors" has led to a profound neglect by governments, policy-makers, public health agencies, the media, and disease associations of how societal "risk conditions" are far more important influences upon health than those individual risk factors. A large problem is that the Canadian public's lack of awareness of the importance of the social determinants of health is not producing any public pressure for these authorities to shift their ways of thinking about health and illness.

A major study illustrates the relative importance for health out-comes of "risk conditions" versus "risk factors." Ontario residents were first asked to describe their health as being excellent, very good, good, fair, or poor. Residents then provided objective evidence of their health status (for example, vision, sight, mobility, pain) that provided each of them with a "functional health" score. These self-reported health scores and functional health scores were related to a number of risk conditions and risk factors.

This study found that, compared to those under 40, those aged 40–64 years have an odds ratio of 1.77 (or 77% greater risk) of having lower functional health scores. Those aged 40–64 years also have more than twice the risk of the youngest group for reporting "fair" or "poor health." For the age 65+ group, the corresponding risks of these adverse health outcomes are almost three times greater for those reporting proof of fair health, and more than three times for poor functional health. Low income, however, leads to an almost four times greater risk of reporting poor or fair health and a two and a half times greater risk of having lower functional health than in the case of high-income individuals. Being of middle income also increases the risk of reporting poor or fair health by 62 percent compared to high-income earners; and it increases the risk of lower functional health by 34 percent as compared to this same higher-income group. Smoking and doing no exercise did increase health risk, but by factors much lower than for the other risk conditions.

Another study provided similar findings. In 2002 Statistics Canada examined the predictors of life expectancy, disability-free life expectancy, and the presence of fair or poor health among residents of 136 regions across Canada.[14] The predictors employed included socio-demographic (or risk condition) factors (the proportion of Aboriginal population, the proportion of visible minority population, the unemployment rate, population size, percentage of population aged sixty-five or over, average income, average number of years of schooling). Also considered in the analysis were the risk factors of rates of daily smoking, obesity, infrequent exercise, heavy drinking, high stress, and depression.

Once again — and consistent with most other research — this study shows that risk behaviours are weak predictors of health status as compared to socio-economic and demographic measures, of which income is a major component. Indeed, the relatively minor health effects of risk factors have been known since the 1970s — a finding confirmed since then by many studies in Canada and elsewhere.

The disproportionate focus on risk factors, then, is misguided. Risk factors are relatively less important to health than are risk conditions; and the emphasis on risk factors has been based on an assumption that all individuals are equally capable of making "healthy lifestyle choices" — with the adjunct that individuals who fail to make these choices are responsible for their own poor health outcomes. Numerous studies have demonstrated that many of the people most vulnerable to disease find it almost impossible to make "healthy lifestyle choices," and that is because they lack the necessary financial resources and are unable therefore to get access to the facilities that would support the required activities.

Evidence also indicates that "healthy lifestyle" programs have little success in benefiting those most at risk for experiencing health problems. The failures of these programs to change risk behaviours or improve health serve only to further discourage those already

Table 1-1. Proportion of Variation in Life Expectancy, Disability-Free Life Expectancy, and Proportion of Citizens Reporting Fair or Poor Health Explained by Different Factors at the Health Region Level in Canada (Total Variation for Each Outcome Measure = 100%)

Predictors	Life Expectancy	Disability-Free Life Expectancy	Fair or Poor Health
Socio-demographic factors only	56%	32%	25%
Additional variation predicted by:			
Daily smoking rate	8%	6%	4%
Obesity rate	1%	5%	10%
Infrequent exercise rate	0%	3%	0%
Heavy drinking rate	1%	3%	1%
High stress rate	0%	0%	1%
Depression rate	0%	8%	9%

Source: M. Shields and S. Tremblay, "The Health of Canada's Communities," *Health Reports — Supplement 13* (July 2002), in D. Raphael (ed.), *Social Determinants of Health: Canadian Perspectives,* second edition, Toronto: Canadian Scholars' Press, 2009.

susceptible to health problems. They also have the potential to create despair and hopelessness among the agencies and workers who administer these "healthy lifestyle choices" programs.

Finally, these approaches have a disturbing tendency to neglect the sources of the difficult living conditions to which many Canadians are exposed, further obscuring the importance of these sources to health. Governments and policy-makers appear at times to be all too eager to attribute health problems to "unhealthy lifestyle choices" rather than to the health-threatening policies that these authorities themselves create.

Despite these problems, the risk factor approach dominates most governmental and public health activity and is the mainstay of disease-association communication. The media reinforce the "healthy lifestyle choices" understandings of the Canadian public

An Example of the Lifestyle Mantra

Eight Healthy Choices to Reduce your Risk for Disease

The big four chronic diseases — cancer, diabetes, cardiovascular disease (heart disease and stroke) and lung disease — are among the most preventable. By making healthier choices, you can lower your risk. You can choose to:

- be a non-smoker and avoid second-hand smoke
- be physically active every day
- eat healthy foods
- achieve a healthy weight
- control your blood pressure
- limit your intake of alcohol
- reduce your stress
- be screened or tested regularly.

Source: Public Health Agency of Canada, "Healthy Living Can Prevent Disease," 2010. <http://www.phac-aspc.gc.ca/cd-mc/healthy_living-vie_saine-eng.php>.

as to the sources of health and illness, making the communication of the alternative approach — the risk condition analysis — almost impossible.[15] Without such understandings, the development and implementation of a health-supporting public policy become far from likely.

What about Medical Research and Health Care?

Since 1900 profound improvements in health status have occurred in industrialized nations, including Canada. Most Canadians believe that we now live longer lives because of greater access to the benefits of medical research and better, more advanced medical care. But despite these important changes, the best estimate is that only 10–15 percent of the increased longevity in the last century is due to improved medical care.[16] For example, the advent of vaccines and similar medical treatments is usually held responsible for the profound declines in mortality from infectious diseases in Canada since 1900. But dramatic declines in mortality had already occurred by the time that Canadians were being given vaccines for diseases such as measles, influenza, and polio and receiving treatments for scarlet fever, typhoid, and diphtheria.

Medical care is certainly important to Canadians, and proper care does much to influence the quality of life of those who are ill. But it does little to prevent disease in the first place.[17] Most analysts conclude that the improvements in health over the past century are due to the changing material conditions of everyday life as experienced by Canadians. The improvements came about in a long list of social determinants: early childhood conditions, education, food processing and availability, health and social services, housing, employment security, and working conditions, among others.

Social Determinants and Public Policy

An array of evidence indicates that an exposure to certain social determinants represents the primary cause of good or poor health and provides the best explanation for the persistent differences in health status among Canadians. These exposures also provide the best explanations for how Canada compares to other nations in over-all health. Canadians generally enjoy better health than Americans, but do not do as well as other nations that develop public policy that strengthens the conditions that make up the social determinants of health.

A number of explanations have been offered to show how the social determinants of health "get under the skin" to influence well-being and cause disease: a "materialist" explanation posits that concrete living conditions — and the social determinants that spring from these living conditions — shape health; a "neo-materialist" explanation extends the materialist analysis by asking how these living conditions come about; and a "psycho-social comparison" explanation considers whether we compare ourselves to others and how these comparisons affect our health and well-being.

At the same time, most approaches to health and disease preven-tion have a non-historical emphasis that fails to take into account the effects upon health of experiences that accumulate over time. Adults, and increasingly adolescents and children, are urged to adopt "healthy lifestyles" to prevent chronic diseases such as heart disease and diabetes, among others. Life-course approaches emphasize that the accumulated effects of experience across the lifespan shape health and the onset of disease, including chronic disease. This perspective directs attention to the impact of the social determinants of health during periods of pregnancy, childhood, adolescence, and adulthood, in both immediately influencing health and providing the basis for health or illness during later stages of life.

Canada's market economy plays its part by determining the distribution of income and wealth through the provision of em-ployment and wages. This distribution plays a large role in shaping whether Canadians are able to gain access to a wide range of social determinants of health such as food, housing, and education, among others.

The market economy — and those who manage and profit from its operation — attempts to move more and more aspects of society into its sphere of operation. The term for this shifting of sectors that historically were considered to be part of the public domain — education, utilities, transportation, health care, housing, and other areas — into the operation of the market economy is "privatization." An associated trend is "commodification," which occurs when resources needed for a healthy life are either privatized or, if provided by governments, must be purchased. When a society provides a resource as a matter of right, the resource is decommodified. In Canada the areas of decommodification have been primarily limited to education from kindergarten to Grade 12, medically necessary procedures, and library services. Among wealthy developed nations, Canada is among those highest in its commodification of what citizens need to be healthy.

The operation of Canada's market economy has been subject to minimal controls. Few restrictions are placed on the ability of businesses to hire and fire, determine workers' levels of wages and benefits, and provide training and advancement to workers. Canada's market economy has also successfully moved formerly public resources such as medical services (for example, screening and lab testing, cleaning services), public resources (Petro Canada and Air Canada) and housing (government-provided social housing and co-ops) into the private domain. In his analysis of the harmful health effects of the market economy's unbridled operation in the United Kingdom, Canada, and United States, British sociologist Graham Scambler calls this form of the market economy "disorganized capitalism." Another apt term comes from sociologist Colin Leys, who talks about "market-driven politics" to explain how this uncontrolled market economy distorts public priorities.[18]

Then too, public policy decisions made by various levels of government will have a strong impact on the various social determinants of health. Much of that impact depends on government decisions about intervening, or not intervening, in the operation of the market economy. For instance, the quality of early life will be shaped by the availability of material resources that ensure educational opportunities and adequate food and housing, among others; these are all areas that can be subject to government intervention. Parents' employment security, wages, the quality of their working conditions, and the availability of quality, regulated child care are other factors. These are conditions or factors that usually do not come under individual control; but they can be adjusted or regulated through public policy decisions made by governments and policy-makers. Each and every social determinant of health has a public policy antecedent that can be modified for better or worse through public policy action.

Why do some nations gather and analyze information about the social determinants of health and use that knowledge to manage the economy and formulate public policy while others do not? Why is there such a gap between knowledge and action on the social determinants of health in Canada? The way a society chooses to provide citizens with various forms of security (such as income, employment, housing, and food security, among others) is revealing. To what extent does Canada's market economy allow citizens to experience the conditions necessary for health? And if the market economy does not meet these needs, to what extent do governments intervene — in the form of public policy — to provide citizens with these conditions?

Social Inequalities

The basket of supports that governments can provide has come to be known as the "welfare state" — a term signifying that governments are using their power to provide citizens with the means to achieve secure, satisfying, and healthy lives. Some critics suggest that Canada's welfare state lags behind that of many other developed nations. If so, this would help explain Canadian policy-makers' apparent resistance to the very concept of social determinants of health.

This book is concerned with the present state of the social determinants of health and how they determine which Canadians stay healthy and which do not. Particularly important is the question of how the operation of the economy and recent policy decisions are either improving or weakening the quality of the social determinants of health in Canada. But the final part of solving this puzzle is to consider the various impacts of these public policy decisions on Canadians who are members of different groups.

Although the social determinants of health influence the health of all Canadians, their effects are especially important for those who are most vulnerable to material and social disadvantage. In Canada, such groups include people on lower incomes and those with lower educational achievement. The people who are at greater social disadvantage also include Canadians of Aboriginal descent, Canadians of colour (especially recent immigrants), women, and persons with disabilities. As the operation of Canada's market economy causes certain social determinants to improve, stagnate, or decline in quality — a process that works in combination with government and policy-maker resistance to intervention through public policy action — it is these Canadians whose health becomes especially subject to risk.

That the more vulnerable Canadians are also the people with lower social status means that they have less power and ability to influence the public policy process. Aboriginal Canadians have less influence than non-Aboriginal Canadians; women have less influence than men; Canadians of colour have less influence than white Canadians; newcomers have less influence than persons born in Canada; those with lower incomes and less wealth have less influence than those with greater incomes and wealth; and persons with disabilities have less influence than those without disabilities. The term that describes these differences in status, influence, and power is "social inequality."

Social inequality, then, is closely related to health inequality. Health inequalities can only be reduced in combination with reductions in social inequalities. But improving health is also about reducing the inequalities in power and influence that exist among

Canadians. Working towards a reduction in health and social inequalities will involve both educating Canadians and building social and political movements in support of a public policy that focuses not just on the social determinants of health but also on a more equitable distribution of resources among the population as a whole.

Notes

1. Interviewed in *Unnatural Causes: Is Inequality Making Us Sick?* 2008. California Newsreel documentary series.

2. J. Mikkonen and D. Raphael, "Social Determinants of Health: The Canadian Facts" <http://thecanadianfacts.org>.

3. Senate of Canada. 2009. *Health Disparities: Unacceptable for a Wealthy Country such as Canada.* <http://tinyurl.com/ye9erpo>.

4. P. Townsend, N. Davidson, and M. Whitehead (eds.). 1992. *Inequalities in Health: The Black Report and the Health Divide.* New York: Penguin.

5. D. Acheson. 1998. *Independent Inquiry into Inequalities in Health.* London: UK Stationary Office.

6. J. Epp. 1986. *Achieving Health for All: A Framework for Health Promotion.* Ottawa: Health and Welfare Canada.

7. CPHA documents on living conditions, public policy and health can be found at <http://www.cpha.ca/en/programs/policy.aspx>.

8. Commission on the Social Determinants of Health. 2008. *Closing the Gap in a Generation: Health Equity through Action on the Social Determinants of Health.* Geneva: World Health Organization.

9. R. Wilkins. 2007. "Mortality by Neighbourhood Income in Urban Canada from 1971 to 2001." Statistics Canada, Health Analysis and Measurement Group (HAMG). HAMG Seminar, and special compilations.

10. R. Wilkins et al. 2000. "The Changing Health Status of Canada's Children." *ISUMA* 1 (2): 47–63.

11. T. Faelker et al. 2000. "Socioeconomic Differences in Childhood Injury: A Population Based Epidemiologic Study in Ontario, Canada." *Injury Prevention* 6: 203–208.

12. G. Davey Smith et al. 2005. "Genetic Epidemiology and Public Health: Hope, Hype, and Future Prospects." *Lancet* 366, 1484–98.

13. S. Nettleton. 1997. "Surveillance, Health Promotion and the Formation of a Risk Identity." In M. Sidell, L. Jones, J. Katz and A. Peberdy (eds.), *Debates and Dilemmas in Promoting Health.* London, UK: Open University

Press; Canadian Population Health Initiative. 2004. *Select Highlights on Public Views of the Determinants of Health.* Ottawa: CPHI.

14. M. Shields and S. Tremblay. 2002. "The Health of Canada's Communities." *Health Reports Supplement* 13 (July): 1–22.

15. M. Gasher et al. 2007. "Spreading the News: Social Determinants of Health Reportage in Canadian Daily Newspapers." *Canadian Journal of Communication* 32 (3): 557–74; M. Hayes et al. 2007. "Telling Stories: News Media, Health Literacy and Public Policy in Canada." *Social Science and Medicine* 54: 445–57.

16. J. McKinlay and S.M. McKinlay. 1987. "Medical Measures and the Decline of Mortality." In H.D. Schwartz (ed.), *Dominant Issues in Medical Sociology.* Second edition. New York: Random House.

17. T. McKeown. 1976. *The Role of Medicine: Dream, Mirage, or Nemesis.* London UK: Neufeld Provincial Hospitals Trust; T. McKeown and R.G. Record. 1975. "An Interpretation of the Decline in Mortality in England and Wales during the Twentieth Century." *Population Studies* 29: 391–422.

18. C. Leys. 2001. *Market-Driven Politics.* London, UK: Verso.

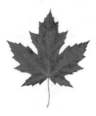

2. LIVING CONDITIONS, STRESS, AND BODIES

> Prolonged stress, or rather the responses it engenders, are known to have deleterious effects on a number of biological systems and to give rise to a number of illnesses. — Robert Evans, health economist, 1994

If risk conditions are the best predictors of health status, and their health effects swamp the influence of risk factors, how, then, do these conditions — our early experiences, the amount of income and wealth available to us, and our exposures to varying quality of employment, food, and housing — come to shape health?

To answer this question we need first to look in more detail at how those social determinants of health get under our skin to create disease and illness. But we also need to take another step back and ask ourselves: Why are there such differences in the living conditions that Canadians experience?"

Getting under the Skin

Much of the prevailing discussion about the social determinants of health falls within a narrow framework: identifying individuals whom health-care providers and health promoters believe are worthy of attention because of their health status and health-threatening behaviours. This approach targets Canadians who experience low-income, insecure and low-wage employment, inadequate housing, food insecurity, and other extremely difficult living conditions, and ideally provides them with appropriate health-care services and risk-factor modification programs. The purpose of these activities is to respond to health-care needs and modify health-related behaviours such as tobacco use, excessive alcohol use, or lack of physical activity.

But these approaches say little if anything about how social determinants themselves directly shape individuals' health or drive their adoption of risk behaviours. These narrow explanations usually do not emphasize actions to alter the makeup of the social determinants of health.

A more useful framework considers how various social determinants directly — and indirectly — influence health, and in particular focuses on how the structures and organization of a society shape the social determinants of health, and health itself (see Figure 2-1).[1]

In this "pathways" explanation, the term "social structure" refers to the organization of a society — its economic system, governments, institutions, agencies, and laws and regulations, and its business, labour, and other interest groups — and how this society distributes material and social resources. The analysis specifically looks at societal decisions that determine how resources are distributed, and considers how these decisions shape the social determinants of health and subsequent health status outcomes.

Three primary "pathways" link social structure with health status (that is, with well-being, morbidity, and mortality. The first pathway is the direct link between material factors and health status. Material factors are the concrete living conditions that include exposure to either health-enhancing or health-threatening situations. These conditions might be related to the quality of housing, diet, and clothing; access to intellectual and emotional stimulation at home, school, and in the community; provision of leisure and recreation facilities; and responsive health and social services.

In the second pathway, the social structure shapes social and work environments to create psychological responses that determine health status. Social environments can differ in their safety and security, their degree of intellectual and emotional support, and their exposure to threats such as crime, family disorder, and role models. Much of these differences in social environments is a result of a governmental willingness to invest in making economic resources available to citizens — resources that provide access to programs and services such as child care, community recreation facilities, public transportation, schools, and social and health services. Social environments shape the material conditions and thus the amount of stress that people experience. These conditions are strong determinants of health.

Figure 2-1. Social Determinants of Health and the Pathways to Health and Illness

The model links social structure to health and disease via material, psycho-social, and behavioural pathways. Genetics, early life, and cultural factors are further important influences upon population health.

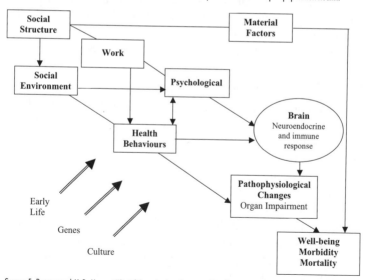

Source: E. Brunner and M.G. Marmot, "Social Organization, Stress, and Health," in M.G. Marmot and R.G. Wilkinson (eds.), *Social Determinants of Health*, Oxford: Oxford University Press, Figure 2.2, p. 9, 2006.

Work environments, for example, differ in a number of ways: their degree of security, the demands made upon workers, and the amount of control that workers have in their workplaces. Work environments also differ greatly in the reward structures that they provide to workers — and these structures are also powerful determinants of health. Again, the differences in work environments are a result of both individuals' employment situations and a governmental willingness to regulate wages, employment conditions, and work environments, and to provide training opportunities. These work environments – like social environments — shape the material conditions and amount of stress that people experience, and thus have a strong influence on health.

The third primary pathway sees these same social and work environments as the keys in shaping behavioural coping responses, such as tobacco use and excessive alcohol use, the adoption of unbalanced diets, such as carbohydrate-rich meals, and sedentary lifestyles that directly impair bodily organs, thereby undermining health. Early life, genes, and culture also contribute to these processes. At all stages of the lifespan, social structure directly influences health.

Material Living Conditions and Health

In one important study, Michaela Benzeval and her colleagues flesh out how childhood experiences influence health not just during childhood but also in adulthood. For them, "income potential" and "health capital" are factors that help to explain how social determinants shape health:

- *Income potential* is the accumulation of abilities, skills and educational experiences in childhood that are important determinants of adult employability and income capacity. Education is seen as the key mediator in this association, being strongly influenced by family circumstances in childhood and a central determinant of an individual's income in adulthood.

- *Health capital* is the accumulation of health resources, both physical and psycho-social, inherited and acquired during the early stages of life which determine current health and future health potential.[2]

In this explanation, the circumstances experienced by children are a result of their parents' characteristics, their objective living conditions, and other aspects of their social environments. These factors all contribute to children's immediate health status and their potential to acquire income in adulthood. Later on, as adults, people will experience health conditions that reflect both their experiences of childhood and their adult situations.

Stress and Health

The human fight or flight reaction evolved as a means of dealing with sudden and dangerous threats in the environment. The body is activated to respond to immediate threats by either fighting or fleeing. That activation involves a number of bodily systems: the sympathetic and parasympathetic nervous systems, the neuroendocrine system, and the metabolic system. After the threat is past, the systems return to their normal levels of functioning.

If the reaction is elicited in a chronic way as a response to continuing threats associated with social conditions such as low income, insecure employment, and housing and food insecurity, among others, the toll on health can be substantial. Chronic elicitation of the fight or flight reaction weakens the immune system and disrupts the neuroendocrine and metabolic systems.[3] Evidence from surveys and explorations of the lived experience of low income, insecure employment, and housing and food insecurity — all social determinants of health — indicate that these experiences make such stress especially likely. Indeed, accumulating evidence shows that individuals who experience constantly difficult or stressful living circumstances come to have maladaptive responses to stress, a

Figure 2-2. The Psycho-biological Stress Response

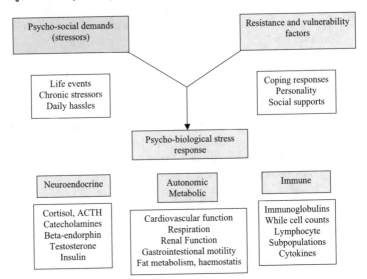

Source: E. Brunner and M.G. Marmot, "Social Organization, Stress, and Health." In M.G. Marmot and R.G. Wilkinson (eds.), *Social Determinants of Health.* Oxford: Oxford University Press, Figure 2.11, p. 27, 2006.

weakened immunity to infections and disease, and a greater likelihood of metabolic disorders.[4]

Health Risk Behaviours and Health

The social determinants of health can also be connected to how people adopt either health-supporting or health-threatening behaviours. For individuals experiencing difficult living conditions and high amounts of stress, "risk behaviours" provide a means of coping. Numerous Canadian studies show that people living under conditions of low income, insecure or no employment, poor housing, and food insecurity are more likely to take up tobacco and excessive alcohol consumption. They will also find it difficult to take up nutritious diets and physical leisure activity.[5]

Similarly, behaviour such as the adoption of carbohydrate-dense diets and weight gain, rather than representing the making of "unhealthy lifestyle choices," represent a coping response to difficult life circumstances. As Mary Shaw and her colleagues at Bristol University put it:

> We also see that some of the factors which contribute to health inequalities — such as smoking and inadequate diet — are themselves strongly influenced by the unequal distribution of income, wealth and life chances in general. These factors do not simply reflect the lack of knowledge or fecklessness of the poorer members of society. If we are to tackle inequalities in health we need an approach which deals with the fundamental causes of such inequalities, not

---

The Lived Experience of Stress

Tracey is a stay-at-home mother of two children. Her husband has a full-time minimum-wage job. She states:

"We fit into the category of 'working poor.' We do not live from paycheque to paycheque — we live from payday to three days after payday, at best. Neither my friends nor my extended family fit into this category, nor do they realize that I do, thus I am constantly struggling to keep up the façade that I am financially okay. The truth is, I'm not. I'm poor. It is degrading and depressing.... I constantly worry about how I'm going to pay the bills, or what I'm going to do if one of our kids get sick and the prescription isn't covered, or what if there is a field trip at school and I don't have the extra money to send my child.... They say that money doesn't buy happiness. But it sure alleviates some of the stress that comes with being poor."

Source: K. Green, *Telling it Like it is: The Realities of Parenting in Poverty* (Saskatoon: Department of Community Health and Epidemiology, University of Saskatchewan, 2001), p. 3.

one which focuses mainly on those processes which mediate between social disadvantage and poor health.[6]

Social Comparison and Health

The "social comparison" approach is usually presented as a competing explanation to the explanations that focus on material living conditions. This explanation downplays the role of the material and social conditions of life in favour of the view that an individual's place in the social hierarchy and "social distance" can explain differences in health status.[7] The argument is that in developed nations people's health status is largely shaped by their interpretations of their standing in the social hierarchy.

This phenomenon occurs on two levels: individually and communally. On the individual level, in unequal societies the perception and experience of lower personal status lead to stress and poor health. When people start to compare their status, possessions, and other life circumstances to the situation of others, they often experience feelings of shame, worthlessness, and envy that have psycho-biological effects upon their health. The comparisons they make lead to attempts to alleviate distress through overspending, taking on additional employment (which can threaten their health), and adopting health-threatening coping behaviours such as overeating and use of alcohol and tobacco. At the communal level, the widening and strengthening of the hierarchy serve to weaken social cohesion and support systems. Individuals become more distrusting and suspicious of others.

This explanation, however, neglects the profound and concrete effects on health of differences in material and social living conditions. The approach is especially problematic in the case of people living in poverty, but it also ignores the growing material insecurity of many middle-class citizens.

The social comparison approach also does not consider political issues: namely, how societal resources are distributed and the political forces that shape these decisions. By stressing psychological processes, it directs attention away from the political, economic, and social forces behind the issues related to the social determinants of health. By stressing the psychological processes of maladaptive coping on the part of people who are experiencing difficult socio-economic conditions, it can lead to "blaming the victim" rather than to a focus on the source of the difficulties.

Still, some of the processes described by the explanation do help to explain how the various social determinants contribute to health status. The act of constantly comparing yourself to others and seeing yourself come up short can clearly lead to health problems. But the source of these comparisons is not in the individual interpretations of the shortcomings, but rather in the social structure and in the processes that create such inequalities. In addition, the perception of coming up short may not originate with individuals who lack resources, but rather with the attitudes and views that exist among societal members who possess a greater amount of resources. These attitudes and views may in turn be shaped by the same societal processes that create and maintain the differing qualities entailed by the social determinants of health, serving to justify the existence of these processes.

Child Is Father (or Mother) — to the Man (or Woman)

The material and social conditions associated with the social determinants of health influence health across the lifespan. Although people often do stop to consider how current living conditions shape health, we also need to recognize the accumulated effects of the social determinants of health throughout life.

Those health effects fall into three categories: latent, pathway, and cumulative.[8] The term "Latent effects" refers to biological and social developmental experiences that early in life have an influence on health later in life. These factors not only have a crucial impact at sensitive periods in human development but also have a lifelong effect regardless of later living conditions. Some of these effects occur during pregnancy and are related to the quality of nutrients that the mother receives, the incidence of infection, and the use of alcohol and tobacco, all of which affect the availability of oxygen to organs. These latent effects come to affect blood clotting and cholesterol metabolism, leading to coronary heart disease and Type II diabetes in later life.

Latent effects upon health can also result from a child's malnutrition and infection during infancy. Malnutrition affects health, cognitive and emotional development, and educational attainment during childhood and later life. Infections can lead to long-term developmental risk and increase problems with airway and respiratory function.

All of these latent effects come into play through the social determinants of health. The incidence of low birth weight, which is a reliable predictor of the incidence of cardiovascular disease and adult-onset diabetes in later life, is one such effect. The likelihood of respiratory problems as an adult is another. An experience of varying nutritional intakes during childhood will have a variety of lasting health effects.[9]

"Pathway effects" are experiences that set individuals on trajectories that eventually come to influence health, well-being, and competence over the life-course. Living conditions, for example, will shape the vocabularies that children have when they enter school.[10] This contingency will set them upon a path that leads to differing educational expectations and achievement, varying employment prospects, greater or lesser accumulation of financial resources, and a differing likelihood of illness and disease across the lifespan. The material and social conditions associated with neighbourhoods, schools, and housing of varying quality also set children on differing paths that either support or threaten health across the lifespan.

Early life may therefore be a particularly important period in itself (a critical or sensitive period), or it may serve as a marker for the path that a person takes through the rest of life. In either event, early life sets most people out on a pathway that leads to the accumulation of exposures that lead in turn to varying health outcomes.

The term "cumulative effects" represents the combination of latent and pathways effects: the accumulation of advantage or disadvantage over time. If children escape disadvantage, the accumulation of disadvantage stops, but the previously accumulated health disadvantage continues with them into adulthood.

How Social Forces Lead to Differing Living Conditions

Given that health outcomes are a result of experiences with social determinants of health of a varying nature over a person's lifespan, we need to extend the analysis to explicitly consider how those living conditions — whether they are an advantage or a threat — come about. Our focus here is on understanding how the social determinants of health result from socio-political decisions concerning how to allocate economic and social resources among the population.

Why is it that in some nations the social determinants of health have an advantageous effect for larger proportions of the population, while in other nations the social determinants lead to a much less satisfactory result, to say the least. And why is it that nations that distribute income and wealth more equitably are also the ones that have higher standards for the delivery of health to their populations?[11]

Canada has a less skewed distribution of income and wealth, and not surprisingly, Canadians generally enjoy better health than Americans as measured by infant mortality rates, life expectancy, and incidence of, and mortality from, a range of diseases and childhood injuries. Still, Canada does not do as well as many European nations in which the distribution of economic and other resources is more equitable and health indicators are more positive. In reality, health indicators in Canada lag behind those of many other developed nations.

In their writings, Canadian health sociologist David Coburn and McGill University social epidemiologist John Lynch illustrate the links between the socio-political resource allocation processes and health determinants.

Coburn argues that when nations allow the market — as opposed to the government regulating the market — to determine the distribution of resources among the population, a resulting deterioration occurs, first in social determinants of health such as income and wealth distribution, and second in the quality of governmental support to citizens in the form of benefits, programs, and services.[12] Lynch also develops this explanation in some detail.

These two would argue that a key social determinant of health, income inequality — that is, the gap between rich and poor — results from a series of processes that reflect decisions within societies to allocate resources inequitably. This process results in increased poverty rates as a direct result of providing low wages and limited benefits to those in need: *individual income for those at the bottom of the social hierarchy*. At the same time, the governments are making only a limited investment in community infrastructure. These limited commitments harm the health of the entire population, but especially those at the bottom of the hierarchy — people who lack the financial resources to purchase the required assets. This explanation directs attention to how income inequality and a lack of investment in various social determinants of health are the result of the adoption by ruling authorities of a neo-liberal ideology, which has an effect on public policy approaches in a variety of areas related to the social determinants of health.

"Neo-liberalism" is the belief that the marketplace should determine how economic and other resources are organized and distributed. It suggests a limited role for government in a wide range of areas. Neo-liberal governments are less likely to take action to strengthen the overall quality of various social determinants of health.

The explanation suggests that whether a nation chooses to strengthen the conditions that make up the social determinants of health is related to a number of factors, such as a nation's history, traditions, institutions, and civic society and culture. The political and economic structures and traditions provide a key to understanding the issue of how Canadians come to experience such differing living conditions. These traditions and the other components — which Lynch places near the top of his explanation — probably also influence how a nation's government responds to another important factor in the area of health: economic globalization.

In his explanation, Coburn outlines how economic globalization is associated with both neo-liberalism and the power of business (for example, in terms of investment decisions) to shape public policy related to the social determinants of health. Business groups can pressure governments to enact public policies that will maximize profits for corporations. These policies may lead to poorer-quality social determinants of health and a more inequitable distribution of these determinants among the population. The policies can lead to lower wages and to government reductions of taxes on corporate and higher

Figure 2-3. A Neo-Material Interpretation of National Approaches to Resource Allocation

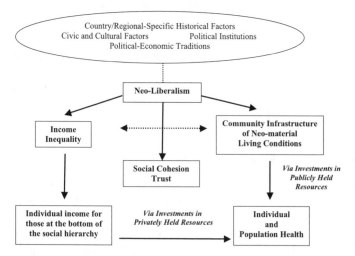

Source: Adapted from J. Lynch, "Income Inequality and Health: Expanding the Debate," Figure 1, p. 1003, *Social Science and Medicine* 51: 1001–1005, 2000.

earners' incomes, which leads in turn to lower government revenues and decreased support for various social determinants of health.

These forces interact with a nation's form of the welfare state and the market. Nations that have developed more equitable-oriented approaches to providing citizens with various forms of security may be more willing to resist these pressures. European nations in general have resisted to a far greater extent than have North American nations the demands of the business sector to deregulate industry and business practices.[13] The amount of resistance to the forces of globalization, neo-liberalism, and private enterprise shapes how these forces play out in a variety of indicators such as income inequality and poverty, and a variety of other social determinants of health. The end result of these public policy approaches is reflected in the quality of health status and well-being as well as in a nation's overall economic wealth. In light of the situation in Canada, Coburn's analysis would suggest that the increasing influence of the corporate elite in Canada has been driving a withdrawal from the traditional Canadian support for the social determinants of health.

It has been suggested that this has indeed been the case with increasing corporate influence being associated with increasing income inequality, consistently high levels of poverty, and stagnating or declining governmental expenditures on various social determinants of health such as education, income, employment, housing, and food security, and health and social services.[14] The mounting weight of evidence appears to support this hypothesis.

Welfare States, Social Determinants of Health, and Bodies

Canadian sociologists Sebastian Saint-Arnaud and Paul Bernard have carefully explored the workings of the economic and political systems and their justifying societal discourses. They provide a narrative that succinctly sums up how these differences in political economy come to be related to the development of differing public policy approaches to promoting health.[15]

Of particular interest are the guiding principles and dominant institutions as they appear in differing welfare states. The United States, Canada, and United Kingdom are liberal welfare states. In a comparative perspective, liberal welfare states provide the least support and security to their citizens. The policy profiles of Canada and the United Kingdom are consistently found to be closer to that of the United States than to European welfare states, where citizen security and support are more ensured.

Within liberal welfare states the dominant ideological inspiration is that of liberty, which leads to minimal government intervention in the workings of the marketplace. Indeed, government interventions are seen as providing a disincentive to work, thereby breeding "welfare dependence." The results of this ideological inspiration are the meagre benefits provided to those on social assistance in the United States, Canada, and United Kingdom, generally weaker legislative support for the labour movement, underdeveloped policies for assisting those with disabilities, and a reluctance to provide universal services and programs. The programs that exist are residual, which means that they exist to provide the most basic needs of the most deprived.

Liberal welfare states and their ideological characteristics would appear to represent the interests of those allied with the central institution of these nations: the market. It is no accident that liberal welfare states have the greatest degree of wealth and income inequality, the weakest safety nets, and poorest performance on indicators of population health such as infant mortality and life expectancy.[16] These states' public policy-makers are seen as being especially responsive to the interests of the business sector, and it is the business sectors in the United States, Canada, and United Kingdom that are most opposed to policies that would reduce social inequality by more equitably distributing income and wealth and strengthening the welfare state through the provision of universal benefits.

Social-democratic welfare states exemplify the opposite situation. The ideological inspiration for the central institution of these nations — the state — is the reduction of poverty, inequality, and unemployment. Rather than seeing government responsibility as being limited to meeting the most basic needs of the most deprived, the organizing principle here is universalism and provision for the social rights of all citizens. Denmark, Finland, Norway, and Sweden are the best exemplars of this form of the welfare state.

Governments with social-democratic political economies are proactive in identifying social problems and issues. They strive to promote citizens' economic and social security. The form of the welfare state has been associated with the virtual elimination of poverty, striving for gender and social class equity, and regulation of the market in the service of citizens. Public-policy action in support of programs that serve to reduce social inequality, such as child-care provision, support for those with disabilities, reducing racism and homophobia, and providing employment training and support for education, among others, is notable.[17]

Even the so-called conservative (Belgium, France, Germany, Netherlands) and Latin (Greece, Italy, Portugal, Spain) welfare states generally provide superior economic and social security to their citizens as compared to liberal welfare states. The ideological inspiration for maintaining social stability, wage stability, and social integration is accomplished through the provision of benefits based on insurance schemes geared to a variety of family and occupational categories. These well-organized benefits schemes are directed towards the primary wage-earners with rather less concern for promoting gender equity than is the case among social-democratic nations.

The "worlds of welfare" typology has been the subject of much debate. Yet no matter what alternative characterizations of the political economy of developed nations are applied, Canada and the United States are always placed in the liberal welfare state groupings.[18] The Scandinavian nations of Finland, Denmark, Sweden, and Norway are almost always identified in the so-named social–democratic realm.

Explicit in some of these frameworks of understanding discussed in these first two chapters — and implicit in others — is that the social determinants of health are shaped by approaches to public policy. The implications of these frameworks are that governments should do whatever they can to strengthen the social determinants of health. In the following chapters we consider a number of these possible approaches.

Notes

1. E. Brunner and M.G. Marmot. 2006. "Social Organization, Stress, and Health." In M.G. Marmot and R.G. Wilkinson (eds.), *Social Determinants of Health.* Second edition. Oxford: Oxford University Press.

2. M. Benzeval et al. 2001. "Income and Health over the Lifecourse: Evidence and Policy Implications." In H. Graham (ed.), *Understanding Health Inequalities.* Buckingham, UK: Open University Press.

3. S. Lupien et al. 2001. "Can Poverty Get under Your Skin? Basal Cortisol Levels and Cognitive Function in Children from Low and High Socioeconomic Status." *Development and Psychopathology* 13: 653–76.

4. D. Raphael. 2007. "The Lived Experience of Poverty." In D. Raphael (ed.), *Poverty and Policy in Canada: Implications for Health and Quality of Life.* Toronto: Canadian Scholars' Press; G. Davey Smith, Y. Ben-Shlomo, and J. Lynch. 2002. "Life Course Approaches to Inequalities in Coronary Heart Disease Risk." In S.A. Stansfeld and M. Marmot (eds.), *Stress and the Heart: Psychosocial Pathways to Coronary Heart Disease.* London, UK: BMJ Books.

5. L. Potvin, L. Richard, and A. Edwards. 2000. "Knowledge of Cardiovascular Disease Risk Factors among the Canadian Population: Relationships with Indicators of Socioeconomic Status." *Canadian Medical Association Journal* 162: S5–S12.

6. M. Shaw et al. 1999. *The Widening Gap: Health Inequalities and Policy in Britain.* Bristol, UK: Policy Press.

7. M. Bartley. 2003. *Understanding Health Inequalities.* Oxford, UK: Polity Press.

8. C. Hertzman and C. Power. 2003. "Health and Human Development: Understandings From Life-Course Research." *Developmental Neuropsychology* 24 (2&3): 719–44.

9. D. Barker. 2001. "Size at Birth and Resilience to Effects of Poor Living Conditions in Adult Life: Longitudinal Study." *BMJ — Clinical*

Research 323 (7324): 1273–76; P.T. James et al. 1997. "Socioeconomic Determinants of Health: The Contribution of Nutrition to Inequalities in Health." *BMJ* 314 (7093): 1545–49.

10. J.D. Willms (ed.). 2002. *Vulnerable Children: Findings from Canada's National Longitudinal Survey*. Edmonton, AB: University of Alberta Press.

11. R.G. Wilkinson and S. Bezruchka. 2002. "Income Inequality and Population Health." *BMJ* 324 (7343): 978.

12. D. Coburn. 2000. "Income Inequality, Social Cohesion and the Health Status of Populations: The Role of Neo-Liberalism." *Social Science & Medicine* 51 (1): 135–46.

13. F. Vandenbroucke. 2002. "Foreword." In G. Esping-Andersen (ed.), *Why We Need a New Welfare State*. New York: Oxford University Press.

14. D. Langille. 2009. "Follow the Money: How Business and Politics Shape Our Health." In D. Raphael (ed.), *Social Determinants of Health: Canadian Perspectives*. Second edition. Toronto: Canadian Scholars' Press.

15. S. Saint-Arnaud and P. Bernard. 2003. "Convergence or Resilience? A Hierarchal Cluster Analysis of the Welfare Regimes in Advanced Countries." *Current Sociology* 51 (5): 499–527.

16. V. Navarro and L. Shi. 2002. "The Political Context of Social Inequalities and Health." In V. Navarro (ed.), *The Political Economy of Social Inequalities: Consequences for Health and Quality of Life*. Amityville, NY: Baywood.

17. G. Esping-Andersen. 2009. *The Unfinished Revolution: Welfare State Adaptation to Women's New Roles*. Cambridge, UK: Polity Press.

18. C. Bambra. 2007. "Going Beyond the Three Worlds of Welfare Capitalism: Regime Theory and Public Health Research." *Journal of Epidemiology and Community Health* 61 (12): 1098–1102.

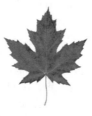

3. FROM INCOME AND EDUCATION TO EMPLOYMENT SECURITY AND WORKING CONDITIONS

Health researchers have demonstrated a clear link between income and socio-economic status and health outcomes, such that longevity and state of health rise with position on the income scales. —Andrew Jackson, Canadian economist, 2009

Four social determinants of health — income, education, employment security, and working conditions — are especially important. They shape the material conditions of daily life, the degree of stress or anxiety experienced, and the extent to which health-damaging coping behaviours are taken up. In addition, since these social determinants influence the amount of economic resources that are available to individuals and families, they also shape the quality of numerous other social determinants of health, such as early child development, food security, housing, and the experience of social exclusion.

A key aspect of the social determinants of health in Canada is that they usually cluster together. Canadians who are advantaged or disadvantaged in one determinant are usually advantaged or disadvantaged in others. In Canada, levels of income and education on the one hand, and employment security and quality of working conditions on the other are strongly related to each other. Much of this has to do with the important role of the employment marketplace in determining the amount of financial and social resources that Canadians can obtain. In a society in which governments hesitate to intervene in the employment marketplace by enacting laws and regulations that would help to ensure employment security, health-sustaining wages and benefits, and adequate working conditions, the quality of these social determinants of health will vary from excellent to very poor. In Canada, such variations in living and working conditions lead to profound inequalities in health outcomes among Canadians.

In Canada employment security, wages, and benefits usually depend more upon a person's personal characteristics, such as social class background and educational attainment, than on workplace laws and regulations. As a result, Canada falls among a group of wealthy developed nations with the highest rates of income inequality and poverty, low-waged workers, and employment insecurity.[1] Canada is also among the most frugal wealthy developed nations in its level of income-related benefits such as family benefits, social assistance levels, and unemployment benefits. All of these factors contribute to inequalities in health outcomes.

Income and Income Distribution

Income is a widely examined — and some argue the most important — social determinant of health. It is usually conceptualized in two differing but related ways. The first way is based on the *actual amount of income* received by an individual or family. This finding provides a discrete measure of economic resources. The analysis then turns to how and why levels of individual and family income come to be so strongly related to health outcomes. The second method is to look at the *distribution of income* across the population. This provides a measure of inequality in economic resources. Inequality describes the gap between rich and poor within a society and provides a context for considering how public policy approaches to income security predict the overall health of a society and the extent of inequalities in health outcomes. Income inequality has proven to be one of the best predictors of the overall health of a society.

The amount of income available to an individual or family is a primary social determinant of health because it shapes overall living conditions, influences psychological functioning, and determines in large part health-related behaviours such as the quality of diet, extent of physical activity, tobacco use, and excessive alcohol use. Income also determines the quality of other social determinants of health such as food security, housing, and other basic prerequisites of health.

Income is especially important in societies that provide fewer important services and benefits as a matter of citizen rights, because these goods then have to be purchased. In Canada, public education until Grade 12, medically necessary procedures, and libraries are funded from general revenues, but child care, housing, post-secondary education, recreational opportunities, and resources for retirement are for the most part commodified: individuals must pay for them. In contrast, many wealthy developed nations provide child care, affordable housing, employment training, and post-secondary education as citizen rights. Public pensions in most other wealthy developed nations are also more generous than they are in Canada.

Individuals and families with lower absolute incomes experience health problems because they face material and social deprivation. The greater the deprivation, the less likely it is that individuals and families can afford the basic prerequisites of health, such as food, clothing, and housing. Deprived Canadians are also socially excluded from participating in the cultural, educational, and recreational activities expected of citizens in an advanced wealthy nation. As we have seen (chapter 2), material and social deprivation causes illness.

Material and social deprivation is a graded phenomenon that cuts across the population to varying degrees from the very poor to the very wealthy. Mary Shaw and her colleagues succinctly described the source of this phenomenon, known as the *social gradient of health*: "The social structure is characterized by a finely graded scale of advantage and disadvantage, with individuals differing in terms of the length and level of their exposure to a particular factor and in terms of the number of factors to which they are exposed."[2]

Just as *income available* is an excellent indicator of the health of individuals and families, *income inequality* is an excellent indicator of the health of the population. As inequality rises, increasing numbers of Canadians are unable to a) have their basic needs met; and b) participate in day-to-day productive and social activities. "Social exclusion" is the term used to describe this process of being "left out" of Canadian life.

Dr. Nathalie Auger and Carolyne Alix of the Quebec Ministry of Health have documented how income is related to health outcomes in Quebec. The patterns they note are illustrative of conditions throughout the country. For example, life expectancy systematically differs as a function of neighbourhood income. In Quebec, men living in the wealthiest 20 percent of neighbourhoods live on average more than four years longer than men in the poorest 20 percent of neighbourhoods. The comparative difference for women in Quebec is just over two years.

Moreover, death rates from a variety of afflictions are also a function of neighbourhood deprivation (calculated as a combination of income, education, and unemployment rates). In terms of death from all causes, those living in the most deprived neighbourhoods had death rates that were 28 percent higher than people in the least deprived neighbourhoods. In terms of respiratory disease, the rates in the most deprived neighbourhoods were 46 percent higher than in the least deprived. Similar findings are shown for deaths from circulatory diseases, accidents, and tumours.[3]

Suicide rates also differ as a function of neighbourhood income. The annual suicide rates in the lowest income neighbourhoods in 2000–04 were almost twice (23.7/100,000) those seen in the wealthiest neighbourhoods (13.0/100,000). Differences were seen in a step-wise progression across five types of neighbourhoods, further illustrating the social gradient of health outcomes related to income differences.

Two Ontario studies illustrate these same income-health patterns. Income is related to the likelihood of suffering from adult-onset diabetes and experiencing first-time heart attacks. One of the studies found that women and men of lower income were much more likely to have diabetes than were wealthier women and men.[4] Low-income women were almost four times more likely to report having diabetes as compared to high-income women. Low-income men were 40 percent more likely to have diabetes than were high-income men.

In the other study, individuals living in lower-income neighbourhoods were more likely to be admitted to hospitals for first-time heart attacks than were those living in wealthier neighbourhoods. The number of admissions for those living in both the poorest and next

Figure 3-1. First-time Heart Attack Admission Rates by Area Income, Ontario, 1994–1997

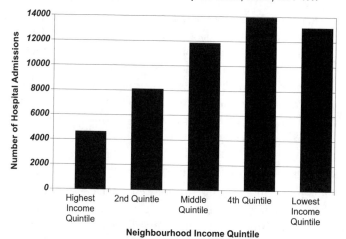

Source: D.A. Alter et al., "Effects of Socioeconomic Status on Access to Invasive Cardiac Procedures and on Mortality After Acute Myocardial Infarction," *NEJM* 341: 1360–67, 1999.

poorest 20 percent of neighbourhoods was almost three times higher than for those living in the wealthiest 20 percent of neighbourhoods. These differences could not be primarily attributed to factors such as being overweight or obese or physically inactive: numerous studies indicate that these differences are a reflection of variations in material and social deprivation and the health outcomes that result from such deprivation.[5]

A Toronto study looked at three key indicators of children's health and well-being as a function of average neighbourhood income: low birth weight for births of a single child (excluding multiple births), readiness to learn at age of school entry, and teen live births. All of these are well-established indicators of both childhood and adult health status and general well-being. For each indicator the health outcomes are worse when the income of the neighbourhood is lower. Additionally, whatever health indicator — for children or adults — one chooses to look at, such profound differences as a function of income are common.[6]

Given that the risk condition of income accounts for these findings rather than the health-related behaviours of tobacco use and physical activity (see chapter 1), our conclusion must be that biomedical and behavioural risk factors provide rather modest contributions to health outcomes when they are compared to income levels and income-related risk conditions.[7] An emerging consensus exists that income inequality and the material and social resources associated with income differences are the key health policy issues that need to be addressed by governments and policy-makers.

The State of Income and Its Distribution in Canada

A 2008 report by the Organisation for Economic Co-operation and Development (OECD) identified Canada as one of two wealthy developed nations (among thirty) that showed the greatest increases in income inequality and poverty from the 1990s to the mid-2000s.[8] The study employed the Gini index, which provides a summary measure of inequality based on a "perfect income equality" coefficient of .00. If one person receives all the income available, the coefficient would be 1.0. Among OECD countries, Canada stands in the middle of the pack. In the mid-1980s Canada's score was .28, which gave it a rank of 11 among 21 nations for which data was available. In the mid-2000s, Canada's score had grown to .32, giving it a rank of 18 of 30 nations.

Ann Curry-Stevens of Portland State University shows that from 1985 to 2005, the bottom 60 percent of Canadian families experienced an actual decline in market incomes in constant dollars, while the top 20 percent of Canadian families did very well. She also shows that increases in income inequality led to a hollowing out of the middle class in Canada, with significant increases from 1980 to 2005 in the percentages of Canadian families who were now either poor or very rich.[9] The percentage of Canadian families who earned middle-level incomes declined from 1980 to 2005, while the percentage of very wealthy Canadians increased, as did those near the bottom of the income distribution.

Figure 3-2. The Majority Loses Ground: Market Incomes for Canadian Families, 1980 and 2005

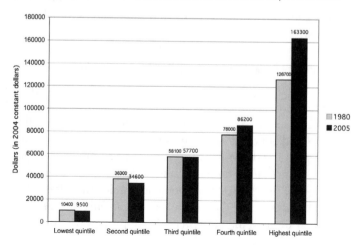

Of even more concern — considering that Canada entered a long recession in 2008 — is Curry-Stevens's finding that income inequality increases dramatically during economic recessions and recoveries. During the recessions of 1981–84 and 1989–93, the market incomes of the bottom 20 percent of Canadians declined by 45 percent and 60 percent respectively while the decline for the top 20 percent of income-earners was .5 percent and 7 percent. However, during recoveries from the two earlier recessions, the bottom 20 percent of income-earners saw their incomes increase by only $2,975 and $1,260 respectively; the corresponding increases for the top 20 percent of income-earners were $14,460 and $12,030.

The increases in wealth inequality in Canada are even more troubling. Wealth is probably a better indicator of long-term health outcomes because it is a more sensitive measure of financial security than is income. Curry-Stevens reports that from the period of 1984 to 2005 the bottom 30 percent of Canadian families had no net worth, and over this period their net worth declined further into debt. In contrast, the net worth of the top 10 percent of Canadian families in 2005 was $1.2 million, an increase of $659,000 in constant dollars from 1984. The next highest 10 percent of families' net worth in 2005 was $400,000, representing an increase of $157,000 from 1984.

The Importance of Public Policy in Shaping Income and Its Distribution

Income and its distribution are strongly shaped by public policy. Governments pass laws and regulations that determine levels not only of minimum wages and employment benefits but also, for those unable to work, unemployment benefits and social assistance rates. Governments also determine income and its distribution by making it easier or more difficult to form unions. Nations that have greater proportions of their workforces belonging to unions have less income inequality and poverty.[10] Governments also influence income and its distribution through the tax system. More progressive tax systems distribute income and wealth more equitably and reduce income insecurity and poverty.

The labour movement influences income and income distribution in numerous ways. Unionized workers earn higher wages and have more benefits than do non-unionized workers. The business community directly influences income distribution through the wages and benefits that it provides employees. It also shapes income and income distribution through its efforts to influence governmental policy-making towards the tax system, labour regulations, and general social policy in a whole range of income-related issues. Business community recommendations concerning these issues tend to lead to greater income and wealth inequalities and increased citizen insecurity.

Recommendations for Improving the Distribution of Income

Anti-poverty groups such as Campaign 2000, Make Poverty History, and the Canadian Association of Food Banks have all put forth recommendations for making the distribution of income more equitable. These organizations urge an increase in the minimum wage and a boost in assistance levels for those unable to work, measures that would provide immediate benefits for people who are at the bottom of the income distribution ladder. They also call for increased child benefits similar to levels provided in other nations.

Another way of reducing income and wealth inequalities would be to make it easier for workplaces to unionize. Creating a fairer tax system would help halt the growth of income inequality in Canada. Tax policy over the past two decades has increased the tax burden of lower- and middle-class Canadians, while reducing the tax burden for the most well-off.[11] In 1990 the total tax burden of the bottom 10 percent of income earners was 25.5 percent of broad income, including market investments and benefits; that figure increased to 30.7 percent in 2005. In contrast, the top 1 percent of earners saw their total taxes being reduced from 34.2 percent to 30.5 percent over the same period; the next highest 4 percent saw a reduction from 36.5 percent to 33.8 percent.

Education and Its Importance for Health

Education is an important social determinant of health. Canadians of higher educational attainment are healthier than are those of lower attainment.[12] An important question is whether it is education that is the cause of better health, or whether education serves as a means of achieving greater material and social resources. There is evidence supporting both arguments. The level of education attained is highly correlated with levels of income, employment security, and better working conditions — all of which are themselves important social determinants of health.[13] Education provides a means by which individuals can move up the socio-economic ladder, which in turn guarantees greater access to health resources and an improved quality of life.

At a societal level, a more educated population should also be a healthier population that is better able to respond to challenges related to the economic and social changes that occur in Canadian society. Being better educated makes it more likely that individuals will be able to benefit from training opportunities within the occupational sphere, and from retraining too, if current employment situations change. Being better educated usually facilitates citizen engagement in the political process in Canada.

Greater literacy is associated with a better understanding of health and its determinants. The field of health literacy is built around the premise that literacy influences the extent to which individuals can promote their own health and those around them. Also, having greater literacy is related to having a greater understanding of the world in general and of how to at least attempt to influence what is going on. The sense of coherence gained has been shown to be strongly related to better health.

Education's relationship to health is strongly embedded in the meaning that educational attainment has within Canadian society. Is education important by itself in attaining better health? Or is it that education is closely connected to other important social determinants of health? As noted in another discussion of the relationship between education and poverty:

> Individual cognitive, social, and educational characteristics associated with specific life trajectories and life experiences by themselves do not lead to poverty. They lead to poverty because they exist within specific Canadian policy contexts that make poverty the likely outcome of their presence. These policy contexts reflect the strong market orientation of Canadian society that shapes the distribution of economic and social resources within the population.[14]

Any analysis of education must also consider how the employment marketplace stratifies individuals on the basis of education and allows those with lesser education to experience health-threatening social conditions. If health-sustaining wages and benefits and necessary services such as affordable child care and housing were available to all, lower educational attainment would in all likelihood become a less important marker of disadvantage in Canada.

The State of Education

Charles Ungerleider of the University of British Columbia and his colleagues point out that Canadian children fare well in international assessments of reading, science, and mathematics achievement; and among the wealthy developed nations of the OECD, Canada has one of the highest proportions (~50%) of its population with some post-secondary education. But these researchers see disparities existing among certain populations and regions, and note that these differences "do not seem to be diminishing with time." They find that lower socio-economic status and second-language students perform less well than students from more advantaged and nonimmigrant backgrounds, though immigrants in Canada fare better than immigrants elsewhere."[15]

Indeed, in an international comparison of achievement ranking, Canada ranked second in science, third in reading, and fourth in mathematics among thirty-six nations participating in testing carried out through the OECD Programme for International Student Testing (PISA).[16] However, as Barbara Ronson and Irving Rootman point out, the OECD's Adult Literacy and Life Skills Survey found that young Canadians whose parents graduated from high school scored twenty-four points better on prose and document literacy than did those whose parents had only eight years of education.[17] In contrast, the situation in Norway saw spreads of only thirteen points for these differing groups of children. Findings like these indicate that nations with well-developed welfare states weaken these parent education–child literacy relationships. Indeed, Swedish children not only outperform all other nations' children in prose, document, and quantitative literacy, but Swedish children whose parents did not complete secondary school usually outperform children from other nations — including Canada — whose parents did complete secondary school.

Recommendations for Improving the Quality of Education

Ungerleider and his colleagues suggest that one means of improving educational outcomes is by supporting early childhood development: "The optimal development of children requires the provision of early, intensive, and, most importantly, systematic early learning programs." [18] Ronson and Rootman propose that governments improve the educational system for young people and develop an effective adult education and training system. Governments should also create policy and funding commitments to ensure that adults have access to a variety of literacy and learning opportunities in their home communities; they should fund projects aimed at increasing the accessibility of information. (For more on the provision of early education resources, see chapter 4.)

Employment and Unemployment, and Their Importance to Health

Employment is a key social determinant of health. Employment provides income and a sense of identity and well-being, and it helps people to structure day-to-day life. When employment is absent, the result is frequently material and social deprivation, psychological stress, and the adoption of health-threatening coping behaviours.[19] The lack of employment is associated with a host of physical and mental health problems that include depression, anxiety, and increased suicide rates.

Employment insecurity has been on the increase in Canada, as Diane-Gabrielle Trembley of the Télè-Université of the Université du Québec à Montréal documents. She noted that at the time of her study in 2006 only about 50 percent of Canadian workers had a single full-time job that had been held for six months or more. Some 14 percent of Canadian workers were self-employed, 10 percent worked temporary jobs, and 18 percent worked part-time; 6 percent had been working in their current employment for less than six months; and 5 percent worked more than one job. Precarious work is associated with greater employment uncertainty, greater stress, and lack of control. All of these are important predictors of adverse health outcomes.[20]

Women are overrepresented in precarious forms of work.[21] While women constitute just over 40 percent of full-time workers, they represent 75 percent of part-time permanent workers and 62 percent of part-time temporary workers. In 1975, 13.6 percent of women were working part-time, and that figure had increased to 27.3 percent by 2000. In contrast in 1975 only 3.6 percent of men were part-time workers — a figure that had increased to 10.3 percent by 2000.

Dr. Emile Tompa of the Institute for Work and Health in Toronto and his colleagues show how the percentage of Canadians engaged in part-time work expanded — and this was particularly the case for the youngest- and oldest-aged groups.[22] They argue that this trend is associated with intensification of work, increased insecurity, and stagnation and polarization of incomes.

Mel Bartley of University College, London, outlines the mechanisms by which unemployment comes to be related to health.[23] The first is that unemployment leads to material deprivation and possibly poverty, which has strong health effects. Unemployment not only reduces income but also removes benefits that were previously available. Both effects are associated with increased likelihood of financial problems. Second, unemployment is a stressful event that is associated with a lowering of self-esteem, a loss of daily structure and routine, and increases in chronic anxiety. Third, unemployment leads to a greater incidence of adverse health-related coping behaviours such as tobacco use and problem drinking.

Insecure employment is usually intensified work and is associated with higher rates of stress, injuries, and back, neck, and shoulder

The Lived Experience of Precarious Work

Vicki Baier enjoyed a comfortable middle-class lifestyle in a small Ontario town until her husband died. Then it got a lot harder to make ends meet. Her job as a cashier with the Liquor Control Board of Ontario (LCBO) did not offer her enough hours to support herself and her sixteen-year-old daughter. Although she had worked there for twelve years, she could not get full-time work, which meant she did not get health or disability benefits. Therefore, when she got breast cancer she had to keep working and arrange treatments during her breaks. Meanwhile, her employer enjoyed sales of $4.1 billion and was able to increase dividends by 5.1 per cent last year. They have clearly profited from the increasing use of casual labour. Vicki is one of over 600,000 part-time and temporary workers in Ontario.

Source: David Langille, *Poor No More: A Film about the Problems and Prospects of the Working Poor*, 2010, <http://tinyurl.com/ykoc8bh>.

pain in individuals. Some studies find that the intensification of work is associated with headaches, sore muscles, fatigue, and nausea. [24]

Non-standard work hours have been related to health issues. Excessive hours of work cause physiological and psychological health problems such as elevated blood pressure and coronary heart disease. Precarious work arrangements are associated with a variety of physical and mental health problems such as stress, anxiety, pain, and fatigue.[25]

One aspect of increasing job insecurity is downsizing, and this process has been associated with increased workplace fatalities, workplace accidents, musculoskeletal injuries, and psychiatric disorders. Perceived job insecurity comes to have negative effects on marital relationships, parenting effectiveness, and children's behaviour.

Recommendations for Improving Employment Security

Job insecurity can be reduced in a number of ways, including through research and education, culture and organizational change, policy and legislation, and reducing inequalities in influence and power. [26]

In the realm of research and education, information should be generated and disseminated that will help to develop new ways of thinking about the health and productivity effects of various management strategies. Strategies that create insecure work may appear to promote competitiveness in the short term, but they can have harmful effects on workers' health and a negative impact on productivity in the longer term. According to the study by Tompa, Polanyi and Foley, "There is a particular need to dispel the assumption that cost-cutting and flexible staffing necessarily lead to economic competitiveness."

In the area of cultural change, both the people within organizations and those outside them have to think differently about work and its effects on health. To develop a new way of thinking about health, Tompa, Polanyi and Foley say, "Workers, employers, government officials, researchers, and others need to come together to develop a shared vision of healthy and productive work."

In institutional change national governments should work to encourage economic pressures that will facilitate the development of "high-road" instead of "low-road" innovation. A long-discussed issue has been the enactment of international agreements that would provide basic standards of employment and work. Rather than a focus on "free trade," perhaps the focus should be on "fair trade."

In the realm of policy and legislation, Tompa and his colleagues argue that nations and companies can work together to develop policy to allocate risk and insecurity among governments, employees, and employers to reduce the health effects of these changes while at the same time enhancing competitiveness: "This can be achieved through a mix of levers such as macroeconomic policy, education and training policy, regulation of workplace practices and benefits, and policies supportive of various forms of worker empowerment through organization and representation."

Finally, there is also a growing power imbalance between employees and employers that must be named and responded to. Inequalities in influence and power exist across differing working groups, and these inequalities need to be addressed. As Tompa, Polanyi and Foley put it: "There is a need, therefore, for stronger legislation governing equal opportunity in hiring, pay, training, and career advancement. Consistent with the notion of reducing inequalities, the requirement of certain accommodations for health conditions would allow freer labour-force participation for older individuals and individuals with functional deficits."

Working Conditions and Their Importance for Health

Andrew Jackson of the Canadian Labour Congress has written extensively about the state of working conditions in Canada — and working conditions are of crucial importance because the experience of work dominates most Canadians' lives.[27] Those Canadians who are already most vulnerable to poor health outcomes due to their lower incomes and education are also the ones most likely to experience adverse working conditions that further threaten their health. The title of Jackson's 2009 analysis — *The Unhealthy Canadian Workplace* — makes the point succinctly.

At the very minimum, work provides people with the necessary income and benefits that profoundly shape the ability to live healthy lives. Jackson identifies a number of work dimensions that shape health outcomes: a) job and employment security; b) physical conditions at work; c) work pace and stress; d) working time; e) opportunities for self-expression and individual development at work, participation in work, and work-life balance

Peter Smith of the Institute for Work and Health in Toronto and Michael Polanyi describe two important ways in which workplace conditions shape health outcomes.[28] The first dynamic, developed by Johann Siegrist, is called "effort-reward imbalance." Research has shown that the degree of incongruence between employee effort in response to demand (for example, time pressures, interruptions, responsibility, pressure to work overtime) and employee reward (monetary, esteem, respect from supervisors and colleagues) is reflected in health problems. When workers perceive that their efforts are not being adequately rewarded, they are more likely to develop a range of illness, afflictions, and problems.

The second dynamic, developed by Robert Karasek, is called "job strain." Jobs can be classified along two dimensions: high control versus low control, and high demand versus low demand. Jobs that are especially related to adverse health outcomes are those in which workers have high demands made upon them but have little control over how these demands can be met. Of the two dimensions, control seems to be the most important: less control is related to more harmful health outcomes.

Most people believe that professional jobs have the highest demands — that professions such as corporate managers, lawyers, teachers, and university professors are the ones most dangerous to health. But unlike working-class jobs, these people have more control over the various ways of coping with the stress — from time management to self-determined vacations. It is the lack of control — which is much more prevalent in working-class jobs — that is the greatest threat to health. As Jackson points out:

> High-stress jobs have been found to be a significant contributing factor to high blood pressure, cardiovascular diseases, mental illness, and long-onset disability. Workers in high-strain jobs are about twice as likely to experience depression as other workers of the same age and socioeconomic status with the same social supports. There is a link between low levels of control over working conditions to stress as well as to higher rates of work injuries. Even where work is physically demanding, there is less risk of injury if workers can vary the pace of work, take breaks when needed, and have some say in the design of workstations.[29]

Other dimensions of the workplace that have been related to health outcomes are organizational justice, work hours, work–life conflict, precarious work, and status inconsistency. All of these dimensions are clearly related to the amount of influence and power that workers have in their workplaces. As such, these conditions are clearly amenable to regulations and laws that would promote greater influence. Unionized workplaces that provide collective agreements are more likely to be able to put such changes into effect.

A great many workers face problems in the form of job security. Jackson argues that the true unemployment rate is probably double the official one. In 2007 the respective figures were 6 percent and 12 percent. Canadians who are unemployed usually cycle in and out of employment. In the same year only 17 percent of unemployed Canadian workers had been out of work for more than six months, while among member nations of the OECD the figure was 47 percent. But precarious work is much more widespread in Canada than elsewhere.

In the European Union, Jackson notes, there is much more effort made to reduce insecurity among workers. In the E.U., job-security laws limit employers' power to lay off long-tenure workers and limit renewals of temporary contracts. Higher minimum-pay levels are mandated, and more widespread collective bargaining leads to higher wages and benefits. In Canada the lack of legislation on these issues leads to far larger pay gaps between precarious and core workers than in most E.U. countries.

The effects of job insecurity are heightened by the difficulty that many people have in getting access to Employment Insurance. Punitive and minimal social assistance programs, according to Jackson, make *any* job look attractive, and the precarious jobs that are available are frequently without benefits such as drug, supplemental health, dental, or pensions. Jackson states: "A large minority of workers experience continuing precarious employment and a significant risk of periodic unemployment. The risks to health of precarious employment caused by stress and anxiety are compounded by lack of access to benefits."[30]

One of the most obvious health–work connections is death and injury at the job. Workplace fatalities continue to be on the increase in Canada, yet reports by workplaces of work-related accidents and injuries appear to be declining. Jackson provides evidence, however, that workplace injuries are seriously underreported because both employers and employees face significant costs in reporting these accidents. While larger unionized workplaces usually emphasize safety, smaller non-unionized workplaces may not. The shift of employment to contracted-out smaller workplaces therefore bodes poorly for preventing workplace injuries.

Jackson also notes apparent increases in repetitive strain and other soft tissue injuries in Canada, along with musculoskeletal pain and chronic back problems. These illnesses take time to appear and workers' compensation programs do a poor job of providing benefits for these types of problems. European Union data provides evidence of increasing intensity of work and declining worker control over the workplace. In terms of Canada, Jackson states:

> Comparable data on the physical demands of work are simply unavailable for Canada, though one recent Canadian survey suggests that the incidence of high speed work in Canada and the US is well above the average of all advanced industrial countries. There is little reason to believe that the situation here is any better than in the E.U.[31]

Unemployment Rates and Job Insecurity

Most Canadians are familiar with the national unemployment rate, which is reported monthly and stood at about 6 percent in 2007. Taken at face value, this number considerably understates the true extent of employment insecurity. To be counted as employed, one need only to have worked for a few hours in a week. Employment figures thus include temporary employees, part-time workers who want more hours, and people working in low-wage survival jobs while looking for regular jobs matching their skills.

To be counted as unemployed, a person has to have been unable to find any work at all, and to have been actively seeking work even if he or she knew that no suitable jobs were available.

Moreover, over a year there is a continual turnover in the ranks of those who are counted as unemployed. While well down from the levels of the early 1990s, a 6 percent average monthly unemployment rate, combined with an average unemployment spell of about twenty weeks, still means that up to 15 percent of the workforce were unemployed at some point in 2007.

Source: A. Jackson, "The Unhealthy Canadian Workplace," In D. Raphael (ed.), *Social Determinants of Health: Canadian Perspectives,* second edition (Toronto: Canadian Scholars' Press) p. 99.

Jackson concludes his analysis by pointing out that 31 percent of Canadian workers believe that their employment puts their health and safety at risk — a figure that is slightly above the average for advanced industrial countries.

Then, too, the jobs that do exist can become particularly stressful when high demands are made on workers but there is little latitude provided on how to accomplish these tasks. Stress from these kinds of jobs is more common among Canadian women than men. Statistics Canada found that 28 percent of women had these kinds of high-strain jobs, as compared to 20 percent of men. These high-strain jobs are more common among low-income sales and services workers.

Statistics Canada also found that in 2000, over one-third of Canadian workers (35 percent) reported experiencing work-related stress from "too many demands or too many hours." This figure is up from a figure of 27.5 percent reported in 1991. Another survey with a somewhat different question found in 2005 that one in three workers (32.4 percent) reported that most days at work were stressful. Women scored higher (37 percent) than did men (32 percent) on an item assessing high-stress levels from "too many hours or too many demands."

With respect to job control, 1994 data found that just four in ten Canadian workers said that they had a lot of freedom regarding work conditions and practices, which Jackson points out is much lower than the 54 percent figure seen in 1989. Men have more control over work (43 percent) than women (38 percent) do, and professionals and managers (51 percent) report more control than do skilled workers (35 percent) and unskilled workers (35 percent). Jackson concludes: "While we lack detailed information on changes in the overall incidence of work involving high demands and low worker control, high-stress work is common and likely on the increase."[32]

Jackson also documents a strong trend to long (and short) working hours for men and women during the 1980s and 1990s. The percentage of men aged 25–54 who work more than fifty hours a week rose from 15 percent in the early 1980s to about 20 percent in 2006, The comparable figures for women are 5 and 7 percent. About 33 percent of men and 12 percent of women now work more than forty-one hours per week. The trend shift to long daily and weekly hours is notably different in Canada and the United States as compared to continental Europe: "The usual weekly hours of full-time paid workers in the EU are below 40, and falling. Some countries, notably France, the Netherlands, and Germany, are now close to a 35-hour norm. The proportion of men working weekly hours much in excess of 40 hours is generally very low.[33]

Recommendations for Improving Working Conditions

Jackson suggests two key areas of action that could be taken to improve working conditions. The first is making more information available about working conditions in Canada. He suggests that Statistics Canada needs to carry out ongoing surveys about working conditions and practices. Without these kinds of information, it is difficult to formulate appropriate responses.

Second, governments must intervene to help shape and improve workplace conditions. He directs attention to numerous recommendations that have been made over the years to improve working conditions. The Donner Task Force (Report of the Advisory Group on Working Time and Redistribution of Work) and the Report of the Collective Reflection on the Changing Workplace called for action not only to "regulate working time by limiting long hours and by making precarious work more secure" but also to implement changes to employment standards and to enhance collective representation of workers.[34]

The report of a federal task force on employment standards, *Fairness at Work: Federal Labour Standards for the 21st Century*, called for "limits on long working-time and arbitrary work schedules, more paid time off the job, and measures to secure respect for human rights in the workplace."[35] Jackson concludes that making it easier for workers to organize is essential because: "It is unlikely that there will be significant positive changes in the workplace if everything is left to employers, and if governments do not help equalize bargaining power between workers and employers."[36]

One way of dealing with a variety of problems associated with working conditions is to equalize the balance between employers and employees. About 30 percent of Canadian workers are members of unions, and the magnitude of differences between unionized and non-unionized workplaces is quite striking. Employees who work under collective agreements negotiated by unions receive numerous benefits and have a greater ability to influence working conditions. Unionized workers covered under collective agreements enjoy higher wages than do those not covered. While benefits are seen across all occupations, the union advantage is especially great for blue-collar and mainly low-wage private services. The union advantage is also especially great for women; in unionized workplaces women earn wages that are 36 percent higher.

Unionized workplaces lead to increased equality of power between employers and employees, greater opportunities for training and advancement, and even greater productivity. Nations with a greater incidence of unionized workplaces also show less income inequality and lower poverty rates, Jackson notes, and the incidence

Table 3-1. Benefits Coverage: Union vs. Non-union

	Medical Plan	Dental Plan-	Life/ Disability Insurance	Pension Plan
All employees	57.4%	53.1%	52.5%	43.3%
Unionized	83.7%	76.3%	78.2%	79.9%
Non-unionized	45.4%	42.6%	40.8%	26.6%

Source: E. Akyeampong, "Unionization and Fringe Benefits," *Perspectives* (August 2002: 3–9). Taken from A. Jackson, "The Impact of Unions," In *Work and Labour in Canada: Critical Issues*, second edition, Table 9.5, Toronto: Canadian Scholars' Press, 2010.

Figure 3.3 Percentage of Low-paid Workers in Canada and Other Wealthy Developed Nations, 2004, 2000*

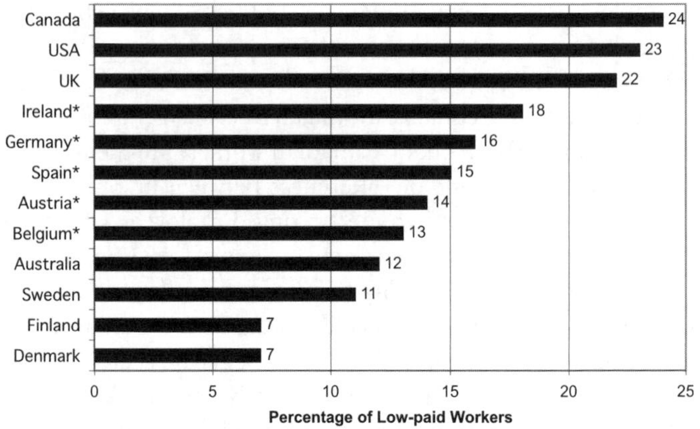

Percentage of Low-paid Workers

Source: S. LaRochelle-Côté and C. Dionne, "International Differences in Low-paid Work." *Perspectives on Labour and Income* June 2009, Ottawa: Statistics Canada.

of lower-paying jobs is less. In 2004 Canada had the highest rates of low-paid workers — defined as earning less than two-thirds of the median national full-time wage — among a number of wealthy developed nations.

More Income and Employment Equality = Better Health

Accumulating evidence indicates that in Canada the quality of these key social determinants of health is either declining or stagnating. While Canadian children do very well in educational achievement, persistent educational attainment differences among groups in Canada remain. Of much more concern is the accumulating evidence of growing income and wealth inequality. Poverty levels remain virtually unchanged from twenty years ago, but the growing inequalities in income and wealth suggest that those already disadvantaged will face even greater challenges in participating in society and maintaining their health than may have been the case in the past.

Additionally, the rise in employment insecurity and evidence of stagnating or worsening working conditions are causes for great concern. Precarious and low-waged employment is on the increase, which can only bode poorly for the future. One way of countering these trends is through the increased unionization of the Canadian workplace and the negotiating of greater numbers of collective agreements.

Much of these developments are related to growing inequalities in power and influence in the employment marketplace and workplace. Average Canadians appear to have less influence with governments and policy-makers than do those at the top of the economic ladder. The result is growing inequality and stagnating wages for most Canadians. If we are to change these conditions, governments must take steps to make it easier for workers to unionize and negotiate collective agreements.

Notes

1. D. Raphael. 2007. "Canadian Public Policy and Poverty in International Perspective." In D. Raphael (ed.), *Poverty and Policy in Canada: Implications for Health and Quality of Life.* Toronto: Canadian Scholars' Press.

2. M. Shaw et al. 1999. *The Widening Gap: Health Inequalities and Policy in Britain.* Bristol, UK: Policy Press.

3. N. Auger and C. Alix. 2009. "Income, Income Distribution, and Health in Canada." In D. Raphael (ed.), *Social Determinants of Health: Canadian Perspectives.* Second edition. Toronto: Canadian Scholars' Press.

4. J. Hux, G. Booth, and A. Laupacis. 2002. *The ICES Practice Atlas: Diabetes in Ontario.* Toronto: Institute for Clinical Evaluative Sciences and the Canadian Diabetes Association.

5. D. Raphael, S. Anstice, and K. Raine. 2003. "The Social Determinants of the Incidence and Management of Type 2 Diabetes Mellitus: Are We Prepared to Rethink our Questions and Redirect our Research Activities?" *Leadership in Health Services* 16: 10–20; D. Raphael and E.S. Farrell. 2002. "Beyond Medicine and Lifestyle: Addressing the Societal

Determinants of Cardiovascular Disease in North America." *Leadership in Health Services* 15: 1–5.

6.   D. McKeown et al. 2008. *The Unequal City: Income and Health Inequalities in Toronto.* Toronto: Toronto Public Health; D. Barker et al. 2001. "Size at Birth and Resilience to Effects of Poor Living Conditions in Adult Life: Longitudinal Study." *BMJ — Clinical Research* 323 (7324): 1273–76; Innocenti Research Centre. 2001. *A League Table of Teenage Births in Rich Nations.* Florence: Innocenti Research Centre; J.D. Willms. 1999. "Quality and Inequality in Children's Literacy: The Effects of Families, Schools and Communities." In D.P. Keating and C. Hertzman (eds.), *Developmental Health and the Wealth of Nations: Social, Biological and Educational Dynamics.* New York: Guilford Press; Canadian Population Health Initiative (CPHI). 2008. *Reducing Gaps in Health: A Focus on Socio-Economic Status in Urban Canada.* Ottawa: CPHI.

7.   G. Davey Smith (ed.). 2003. *Inequalities in Health: Life Course Perspectives.* Bristol UK: Policy Press; M. Shaw et al. 1999. *The Widening Gap: Health Inequalities and Policy in Britain.* Bristol, UK: Policy Press.

8.   Organisation for Economic Co-operation and Development (OECD). 2008. *Growing Unequal: Income Distribution and Poverty in OECD Nations.* Paris: OECD.

9.   A. Curry-Stevens. 2009. "When Economic Growth Doesn't Trickle Down: The Wage Dimensions of Income Polarization," In D. Raphael (ed.), *Social Determinants of Health: Canadian Perspectives.* Second edition. Toronto: Canadian Scholars' Press.

10.   D. Raphael. 2009. "Reducing Social and Health Inequalities Requires Building Social and Political Movements." *Humanity and Society* 33, (1/2): 145–65.

11.   M. Lee. (2007). *Eroding Tax Fairness: Tax Incidence in Canada, 1998 to 2005.* Ottawa: Canadian Centre for Policy Alternatives.

12.   Canadian Population Health Initiative (CPHI). 2004. *Improving the Health of Canadians.* Ottawa: CPHI.

13.   B. Ronson and I. Rootman. 2009. "Literacy and Health Literacy: New Understandings about their Impact on Health." In D. Raphael (ed.), *Social Determinants of Health: Canadian Perspectives.* Second edition. Toronto: Canadian Scholars' Press; C. Ungerleider, T. Burns, and F. Cartwright. 2009. "The State and Quality of Canadian Public Elementary and Secondary Education." In D. Raphael (ed.), *Social Determinants of Health: Canadian Perspectives.* Second edition. Toronto: Canadian Scholars' Press.

14. D. Raphael. 2007. *Poverty and Policy in Canada: Implications for Health and Quality of Life*. Toronto: Canadian Scholars' Press.

15. C. Ungerleider, T. Burns, and F. Cartweight. 2009. "The State and Quality of Canadian Public Elementary and Secondary Education." In D. Raphael (ed.), *Social Determinants of Health: Canadian Perspectives*. Second edition. Toronto: Canadian Scholars' Press.

16. PISA database <http://pisa2006.acer.edu.au/>; Publication: PISA 2006 Science Competencies for Tomorrow's World.

17. B. Ronson and I. Rootman. 2009. "Literacy and Health Literacy: New Understandings about their Impact on Health." In D. Raphael (ed.), *Social Determinants of Health: Canadian Perspectives*. Second edition. Toronto: Canadian Scholars' Press.

18. C. Ungerleider, T. Burns, and F. Cartweight. 2009. "The State and Quality of Canadian Public Elementary and Secondary Education." In D. Raphael (ed.), *Social Determinants of Health: Canadian Perspectives*. Second edition. Toronto: Canadian Scholars' Press.

19. M. Bartley. 1994. "Unemployment and Ill Health: Understanding the Relationship." *Journal of Epidemiology and Community Health* 48: 333–37.

20. W. Lewchuk et al. 2006. "The Hidden Costs of Precarious Employment: Health and the Employment Relationship." In L. Vosko (ed.), *Precarious Work in Canada*. Kingston: McGill Queen's University Press.

21. D.G. Tremblay. 2009. "Precarious Work and the Labour Market." In D. Raphael (ed.), *Social Determinants of Health: Canadian Perspectives*. Second edition. Toronto: Canadian Scholars' Press.

22. E. Tompa, M. Polanyi, and J. Foley. 2009. "Labour Market Flexibility and Worker Insecurity." In D. Raphael (ed.), *Social Determinants of Health: Canadian Perspectives*. Second edition. Toronto: Canadian Scholars' Press.

23. M. Bartley. 1994. "Unemployment and Ill Health: Understanding the Relationship." *Journal of Epidemiology and Community Health* 48: 333–37.

24. E. Tompa, M. Polanyi, and J. Foley. 2009.

25. W. Lewchuk, M. Clarke, and A. de Wolff. 2008. "Working without Commitments: Precarious Employment and Health." *Work Employment Society* 22 (3): 387–406.

26. E. Tompa, M. Polanyi, and J. Foley. 2009.

27. A. Jackson. 2005. *Work and Labour in Canada: Critical Issues*. Toronto: Canadian Scholars' Press; A. Jackson. 2009. "The Unhealthy Canadian Workplace." In D. Raphael (ed.), *Social Determinants of Health: Canadian Perspectives*. Second edition. Toronto: Canadian Scholars' Press.

28. P. Smith and M. Polanyi. 2009. "Understanding and Improving the Health of Work." In D. Raphael (ed.), *Social Determinants of Health: Canadian Perspectives.* Second edition. Toronto: Canadian Scholars' Press.

29. A. Jackson. 2009. "The Unhealthy Canadian Workplace." In D. Raphael (ed.), *Social Determinants of Health: Canadian Perspectives.* Second edition. Toronto: Canadian Scholars' Press.

30. A. Jackson. 2009. "The Unhealthy Canadian Workplace." In D. Raphael (ed.), *Social Determinants of Health: Canadian Perspectives.* Second edition. Toronto: Canadian Scholars' Press: p. 103.

31. A. Jackson. 2009. "The Unhealthy Canadian Workplace." In D. Raphael (ed.), *Social Determinants of Health: Canadian Perspectives.* Second edition. Toronto: Canadian Scholars' Press: p. 106.

32. A. Jackson. 2009. "The Unhealthy Canadian Workplace." In D. Raphael (ed.), *Social Determinants of Health: Canadian Perspectives.* Second edition. Toronto: Canadian Scholars' Press: p. 107.

33. A. Jackson. 2009. "The Unhealthy Canadian Workplace." In D. Raphael (ed.), *Social Determinants of Health: Canadian Perspectives.* Second edition. Toronto: Canadian Scholars' Press: p. 108.

34. Canada. 1994. Advisory Group on Working Time and the Distribution of Work. *Report of the Advisory Group on Working Time and the Distribution of Work.* Hull, PQ: Human Resources and Development Canada; Canada. 1997. *Report of the Collective Reflection on the Changing Workplace.* Hull, PQ: Human Resources and Development Canada

35. Human Resources and Skills Development Canada (HRSD). 2006. *Fairness at Work: Federal Labour Standards for the 21st Century.* Ottawa: HRSD Canada.

36. A. Jackson. 2009. "The Unhealthy Canadian Workplace." In D. Raphael (ed.), *Social Determinants of Health: Canadian Perspectives.* Second edition. Toronto: Canadian Scholars' Press: p. 112.

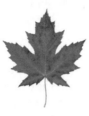

4. EARLY CHILD DEVELOPMENT, FOOD SECURITY, AND HOUSING

> There is strong evidence that early childhood experiences influence coping skills, resistance to health problems and overall health and well-being for the rest of one's life. — Federal/Provincial Territorial Advisory Committee on Population Health, *Report on the Health of Canadians*, 1996

We know, then, that the quality of health determinants are strongly related to the amount of income that people receive. But the quality of these social determinants is also strongly shaped, for better or worse, by specific governmental policies. For instance, the quality of early child development — a strong determinant of health — is significantly influenced by the family benefits and subsidies provided by governments, and also by the provision of affordable high-quality early child education and care, or lack thereof.[1]

The quality of housing that people attain is also influenced by the amount of income available; but, again, another key to good housing is the governmental policies that regulate rents, require the construction of affordable housing, or provide affordable housing according to need. Similarly, food security is influenced not just by income levels, but by food policy and other public policies that have an effect on the affordability of housing.

These three social determinants are fundamental to health and directly amenable to public policy. The establishing of conditions to support healthy childhoods, provide adequate housing, and ensure the availability of adequate food, has also been the subject of numerous human rights covenants and agreements — all signed by Canadian governments — that require governments to provide for these needs as basic human rights.[2] The relationship among these determinants is illustrated by the dilemma that many Canadians face of whether to "pay the rent or feed the kids." For each of these social determinants of health the evidence indicates that the current situation in Canada is not conducive to good health outcomes; predictable adverse health outcomes are associated with the prevailing situation; and Canada is lagging far behind other nations in addressing these issues.

Early Child Development and Its Importance to Health

Viewing early child development as a social determinant of health recognizes that experiences during the beginnings of the lifespan have strong effects upon health. These experiences are both "immediate" — shaping young children's health — and "long-lasting" — providing the foundations for either good or poor health during later periods of the lifespan. The quality of early child development is shaped by the economic and social resources available to parents and the extent to which governments provide a range of supports and benefits to families and their children.

Early child development is important, first of all, because the experiences of early childhood can produce long-lasting biological, psychological, and social effects that determine health later in life: the latency effects. Second, the experiences of early childhood set children off on particular trajectories that lead to later experiences that determine heath: the pathway effects. Third, the experiences of early childhood accumulate, so that the longer the exposure to positive experiences the better the later health outcomes.[3] Conversely, the longer the exposures to adverse experiences, the worse the later outcomes will be.

"Biological embeddedness" refers to how specific experiences come to have long-lasting effects upon health and developmental outcomes.[4] Clear evidence — based on studies that follow individuals over time — indicates that early childhood and even pre-birth experiences predispose children to either good or poor health regardless of later life circumstances. But all is not determined by early childhood experiences. Among the people in a position of socio-economic advantage — whose offspring first of all are less likely to be of lower birth weight — low birth-weight children are much less likely to show these health problems.[5]

These latency effects result from biological processes that occur during pregnancy — processes associated with a poor maternal diet, parental risk behaviours, or an experience of stress. Early childhood experiences such as the experience of numerous infections or the impacts of adverse housing conditions can also have health effects later in life regardless of the circumstances in those years. The traumas of early experience can also lead to psychological health-related problems in later life; as in the case of workplace conditions, a sense of control or self-efficacy has been found to be an important determinant of health.[6]

At one point children's exposures to adverse living conditions may not have immediate health effects, but they can lead to situations that do have health consequences. An important instance of this would be young children's lack of readiness to learn as they enter school. This by itself is not necessarily a health issue, but it leads to experiences that later on do clearly have an impact on health. A lack of school readiness — itself strongly related to family income — leads to lower educational and employment attainments.[7] These lower attainments lead to lower-quality and more insecure employment. These difficult employment situations are important predictors of poor health outcomes.

School readiness is therefore both a result of the social determinants of parents' income and educational status as well as a predictor of their children's later income and educational status. One way of interrupting this sequence is to weaken the relationship between parents' income and educational status and children's developmental outcomes through the provision of high-quality early child education.

Many nations have taken steps towards this goal. Research by Douglas Willms of the University of New Brunswick reveals that the link between socio-economic position and developmental outcomes is weaker in nations with well-developed early child education programs.[8] In Canada these relationships are so important that, as Robert Evans, Clyde Hertzman, and Steven Morgan of the University of British Columbia argue, the establishment of a comprehensive early child education program in Canada would be the single best means of improving Canadian health outcomes.[9]

Cumulative effects are illustrated by findings that the longer children live under conditions of material and social deprivation, the more likely they are to experience health and developmental problems — physical and mental health illnesses and cognitive and emotional deficits such as social and emotional immaturity. The accumulation of difficult experiences during early childhood predisposes children towards a state of learned helplessness, in which they feel unable to act effectively upon their world. Such helplessness is a strong determinant of health in general and a precursor of the adoption of health-threatening behaviours.

Hertzman and Chris Power suggest that the policy response provided by the latency argument is to intervene, and "the earlier the better." The message of the pathways view is "to intervene at strategic points in time." The suggestion of the cumulative model is to "intervene wherever there is an effective intervention."[10]

The State of Early Child Development

In Canada the state of early child development is cause for concern. The most obvious indicator of whether a problem exists or not is the extent to which children are living under conditions of material and social deprivation; and the best measure of this possibility is the percentage of children living in "straitened living circumstances" or below Statistic Canada's low-income cut-offs (LICOs). LICOs identify Canadians who are spending significantly more resources on the necessities of housing, clothing, and food than the average.[11]

The child poverty figure of 15 percent provided by Statistics Canada's pre-tax LICO is identical to figures provided by international organizations such as the OECD and the Innocenti Research Centre of the United Nations International Children Emergency Fund.[12] These organizations define child poverty as the state of living in families that have access to less than 50 percent of the median family income of that nation. In these comparisons, 15 percent of Canadian children are living in poverty, which gives Canada a rank of twentieth among thirty wealthy developed nations.

In an international study that examined whether nations are meeting various early childhood development objectives, Canada ranked as last — tied with Ireland — of twenty-five wealthy developed nations in meeting internationally applicable benchmarks for early child care and education.[13] The report describes these benchmarks as a "set of minimum standards for protecting the rights of children in their most vulnerable and formative years" (p. 2). Canada meets one of the ten standards. Considering that only 17 percent of Canadian families have access to regulated child care, these findings are not surprising. Importantly, the report shows that the nations meeting the greatest number of benchmarks have the lowest infant mortality and lowest low birth-weight rates.

Early child development is influenced by governmental support of families, the strength of the labour movement, and the business community's willingness to provide a living wage. But Canada is increasingly being recognized as a "child-unfriendly" nation. The government, as the international study makes clear, has failed to meet early child education and care goals. That the country has one of the highest proportions of children living in poverty is largely due to the high proportions of low-paid workers: Canada's minimum wages, replacement benefits during unemployment, and social assistance benefits are amongst the lowest of the wealthy nations.

Among those whose workplaces are covered by union-negotiated collective agreements, the income situation is somewhat better; but, only about 30 percent of Canadians workers are covered by union-negotiated agreements. Union density and the presence of collective agreements are important correlates of child poverty. In nations with strong union memberships, child poverty rates are much lower. Continental workers benefit by working under collective agreements that are negotiated between employer association and unions. Nations with lower union membership and lack of such collective agreement show the highest child poverty rates.

Important segments of the business community in the form of some of its largest and most influential organizations have been strong opponents of increasing the wages and benefits available to families with children. To give just one example, in a brief presented to the Newfoundland and Labrador 2008 Minimum Wage Review, the Newfoundland and Labrador Business Coalition, made up of members of a variety of different business sectors, opposed the provincial government's proposal to raise the minimum wage to $10 an hour.[14]

Similarly, through their strong — and mostly successful — efforts to reduce the extent of governmental tax revenues, business organizations — together with conservative organizations such as the Canadian Taxpayers Federation and the Fraser and C.D. Howe institutes — have made it difficult for governments to support families with children through the provision of family-related benefits and early child education and care programs.

Recommendations for Improving the Quality of Early Childhood Education

An improvement in the quality of early child development would have health repercussions for Canadians across the socio-economic spectrum, from the most vulnerable members of society to well-off Canadians, who would benefit through a better quality of life in their communities, reduced social problems, and enhanced Canadian economic performance.

Proposals for improving early child development are virtually the same as those for reducing poverty in general and child poverty in particular. Not only are these recommendations similar to those of other Canadian policy organizations, but they are also similar to the policy directions that have been effective in bettering the early child development in wealthy industrial nations.[15]

Food Security and Its Importance for Health

Food insecurity is about people — including large numbers of children — going hungry, and this in a relatively rich country that can certainly afford to provide all of its population with the nutrition necessary to lead healthy lives. Food insecurity is about uncertainty — in technical terms, about "the inability to acquire or consume an adequate diet quality or sufficient quantity of food in socially acceptable ways, or the uncertainty that one will be able to do so."[16] Food security is a huge issue in Canada. As University of Calgary nutrition professor Lynn McIntyre and research associate Krista Rondeau put it, "A very brief social history of food insecurity in Canada would read simply: Poverty increased, then it deepened. Food insecurity emerged, then it increased in severity."[17]

In a 2004 national survey, Statistics Canada found that an estimated 9.2 percent of Canadian households were experiencing food insecurity.[18] If this kind of finding seems abstract, consider one of the statements that Health Canada used in its measurement of food insecurity: "You and other members of your household worried that food would run out before you got money to buy more." Another tangible indicator of food insecurity has been the appearance and growth of food banks in Canada since the mid-1980s. In March 2009, for instance, 794,738 Canadians made use of food banks — and 37 percent of these "clients" were children.[19]

Whether adults or children, people who suffer from food insecurity are simply not getting as many servings of fruits and vegetables and milk products compared to people in food-secure households. They are getting significantly less minerals and vitamins — falling below the daily requirements for protein, vitamins A and C, thiamine, riboflavin, vitamin B6 and B12, folate, magnesium, phosphorous, and zinc; they do not meet current nutrient requirements as outlined by Agriculture Canada.[20] University of Toronto nutrition professor Tarasuk concludes: "Household food insecurity poses a very real threat to the nutritional status of adults and adolescents."[21]

The dietary deficiencies of food-insecure households contribute to an increased likelihood of chronic disease as well as difficulties in managing these diseases. Canadians are well aware that a healthy diet contributes to chronic disease prevention and the management of these chronic diseases when they do occur, which is especially relevant in cases of diabetes and cardiovascular disease. Yet individuals in food-insecure households are more likely to report the presence of heart disease, diabetes, high blood pressure, and food allergies that persist even when factors such as age, sex, income adequacy, and education are taken into account.[22] In addition, household food insecurity has been shown to have a direct correspondence with whether or not Canadians report poor or fair health as compared to good, very good, or excellent health; and whether they experience poor functional health (pain, hearing and vision problems, restricted mobility), multiple chronic conditions, and major depression or distress.

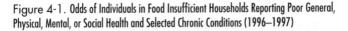

Figure 4-1. Odds of Individuals in Food Insufficient Households Reporting Poor General, Physical, Mental, or Social Health and Selected Chronic Conditions (1996–1997)

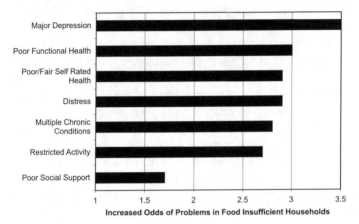

Source: N. Vozoris and V. Tarasuk, "Household Food Insufficiency is Associated with Poorer Health," *Journal of Nutrition* 133: 120–27, 2003.

Finally, increasing numbers of studies indicate that children in food-insecure households are more likely to experience a whole range of behavioural, emotional, and academic problems than are children living in food-secure households. Tarasuk suggests that while families appear to be protecting their children from the nutritional effects of food insecurity — studies show that mothers cut back on their own food intakes to allow their children to have an adequate diet — "It would appear that they are less successful in protecting their children from the negative psychological impacts of household food insecurity."[23]

The State of Food Security

In 2004 over 1.1 million Canadian households — some 2.7 million Canadians in all, or 8.8 percent of the total population — experienced food insecurity. If we look only at families with children, the figures from the same year show that 5.2 percent of them reported child-level food insecurity. Even though this particular survey did not include Aboriginals living on reserves, 33.4 percent of Aboriginal households living off-reserve suffered from food insecurity.

Once again, contrary to popular opinion as disseminated in the news media and in the world of healthy lifestyles promotion, food insecurity is not due to any basic lack of knowledge, poor budgeting, or other personal deficiency on the part of the families that experience this problem. The cause of food insecurity is no secret, and is not at all complicated: it is directly related to the level of household income — it is simply a matter of families lacking the financial resources necessary to maintain healthy diets on a daily basis. The families that are most likely to experience food insecurity are the families that are economically deprived. A 1994 survey showed that lone female-led families were eight times more likely than other families to report their children going hungry, and that trend has not changed in the years since that survey was carried out. When a lone-parent, female-led family receives social assistance, the members became no better off: those families are thirteen times more likely to report their children going hungry. A 1996 analysis found that the likelihood of hunger among Canadian families increased as a function of a mother reporting fair or poor health (fourfold greater risk), the family being led by a lone parent (threefold greater risk), and the family being of Aboriginal status (60 percent greater risk). Even in wealthy Alberta, with its booming oil economy, conditions are critical: a 2004 Community Health Survey found that 84 percent of Alberta households receiving social assistance were experiencing food insecurity, the highest rate in Canada.[24]

The causes of food insecurity therefore lie in governmental and business-sector reluctance to provide Canadian families with the economic resources necessary for health. The solutions to the problem of food insecurity fall back on the same public policies required to reduce poverty.

Recommendations for Improving Food Security in Canada

If public policy is to fully address food insecurity, the first item on the agenda must be to ensure an increase in the incomes of those experiencing food insecurity, which means, as a start, legislating increased minimum wages or social assistance rates. Governments must also make sure that healthy foods, especially staples such as milk, are affordable. As McIntyre and Rondeau assert: "Community-based food-assistance programs such as food banks do not support the achievement of healthy diets among recipients. These initiatives represent a poor policy alternative to the family purchase of healthy foods."[25]

The availability of affordable housing has to be a key governmental priority. Too often families are forced to decide between paying the rent or feeding the kids. A lack of affordable child care is another barrier that often keeps mothers out of the workforce: a universal, publicly funded (which means affordable) child-care system must be set in place.

Finally, governments should expand on programs that have been shown to reduce poverty and food insecurity, providing an integrated slate of work-related supports, health and recreation provision, and other transition assistance.

Housing, Homelessness, and Health

The link between inadequate housing and adverse health outcomes was a key component of Friedrich Engel's 1845 analysis of the *Condition of the Working Class in England.* Almost a century and a half later, in 1986, the World Health Organization recognized shelter as a prerequisite for health.[26] Since then numerous studies have shown that housing quality is an important determinant of health. Indeed, it is an absolute necessity: the evidence indicates that increasing housing insecurity and especially homelessness in Canada are clear threats to health.

The presence of a housing crisis in Canada is particularly

noticeable in the increasing numbers of Canadians experiencing homelessness and housing insecurity — an issue so apparent that it has received the attention of the international community. Like food insecurity, housing quality and housing insecurity are strongly related to the availability of economic resources for families and individuals: a Canada Mortgage and Housing Corporation and Statistics Canada study on housing conditions in Census metropolitan areas between 1991 and 2001 found that the main issue for most households was finding affordable housing, particularly for households that rent.[27] These conditions — of housing and housing security — are also strongly related to public policy because governments have traditionally concerned themselves with meeting the housing and shelter needs of citizens. Yet despite this evidence and the growing housing crisis in Canada, the various levels of government have made only a meagre effort to address this issue. That Canada appears to be sadly failing in meeting its obligations on the housing front is great cause for concern.

International Attention to Canada's Housing Crisis

"Everywhere that I visited in Canada, I met people who are homeless and living in inadequate and insecure housing conditions. On this mission I heard of hundreds of people who have died, as a direct result of Canada's nation-wide housing crisis. In its most recent periodic review of Canada's compliance with the International Covenant on Economic, Social and Cultural Rights, the United Nations used strong language to label housing and homelessness and inadequate housing as a 'national emergency.' Everything that I witnessed on this mission confirms the deep and devastating impact of this national crisis on the lives of women, youth, children and men."

Source: Miloon Kothari, "Preliminary Observations of Mission to Canada," United Nations: Special Rapporteur on the Right to Adequate Housing, 2007.

Why Housing Is Important to Health

Having shelter from the elements is absolutely essential to a humane existence. Even when shelter is achieved, its quality has profound effects upon health. One would think that the prevailing conditions — that on any given day thousands of Canadians are without decent shelter, and hundreds of thousands are living in insecure living conditions — would be cause for concern and action on the part of Canadian governments and policy-makers. Sadly, the housing crisis in Canada appears to receive as much public policy attention as does the food insecurity crisis, that is, hardly any.

Housing is tightly connected to health in a number of ways. First, the proper quality of housing provides individuals with qualitatively different material environments in which they are able to carry out their lives. Second, good housing provides a platform for self-identity and self-expression. And third, the issue of housing has a serious ripple effect: when people have to spend excessive amounts of their income on housing they will have less money left over to manage the expenses related to other social determinants of health.[28]

One extensive review of housing and health research provided stark evidence of the connection between adverse living circumstances and a range of health issues. The study's "definitive findings" revealed "health effects associated with the presence of lead, asbestos, poor heating systems, and lack of smoke detectors." The study also noted the "presence of radon, house dust mites, cockroaches, and cold and heat" — all factors contributing to health problems among residents. The list went on, with "strong findings" seen "for environmental tobacco smoke. Possible findings were seen for dampness and mould, high-rise structures, overcrowding and high density, poor ventilation, and poor housing satisfaction."[29]

U.K. studies revealed similar connections. One case explored how heating and dampness influence health. For example, one-quarter of those surveyed said they were unable to afford as much heat as they would have preferred. Another study found that dampness was contributing to respiratory illness and making it worse: it found, among children living in homes with damp and mould in Edinburgh, an increased risk of wheezing and chesty coughs. Another saw an increased risk of various symptoms of respiratory illness for both children and adults in damp and mouldy houses as compared to those living in dry dwellings.[30]

But, as health studies professor Toba Bryant of the University of Toronto points out: "It is difficult to separate the effects of any single variable or sets of variables upon health [because] indicators of disadvantage — poverty, poor housing, pre-existing illness — frequently cluster together."[31] Still, one such study — *Home Sweet Home: The Impact of Poor Housing on Health* — was, with a very large sample examined over time, able to get around this problem. The researchers showed how adverse living conditions predicted problematic health outcomes among more than 13,000 citizens.[32] Poor housing conditions during childhood played a significant and independent role in determining health outcomes: the worse the conditions, the greater the likelihood of severe or moderate ill health at age thirty-three.

Children who experienced overcrowded housing conditions up to age eleven had a higher likelihood of infectious disease as adults. In adulthood, conditions of overcrowding increased the likelihood of respiratory disease. The experience of living in poor housing in either the past or the present made independent contributions to the likelihood of poor health. The worse situation was to have lived in adverse housing in both the past and the present. Another U.K. study found that adverse housing conditions during childhood predicted early death in selected parts of the country: associations were found between the lack of a private indoor tapped water supply and increased mortality from coronary heart disease, and between poor ventilation and overall mortality.[33]

The most drastic housing connection to health is homelessness. Homeless people are much more likely to experience numerous physical and mental health problems than the members of the general population. Homeless people experience very high levels of respiratory disease, alcohol and drug dependence, and mental health problems; and they are prone to suicide, accidents, and violence.[34]

A Toronto survey of homeless people, for example, found a much higher risk than in the general population for chronic respiratory diseases, arthritis or rheumatism, hypertension, asthma, epilepsy, and diabetes. Similarly, homeless people die at a younger age than do people in the general population: a Toronto study found that between 1979 and 1990, 71 percent of homeless people who died were younger than seventy years. The corresponding figure for the general population was 38 percent. Dr. Stephen Hwang of St. Michael's Hospital in Toronto found in a survey of 9,000 men who used shelters in 1995 that they were eight times more likely to die than were men in the general population. Still another study found that among homeless people in Toronto, death rates were a very high 515 per 100,000 person-years for homeless women aged 18–44 years and 438 per 100,000 person-years for homeless women aged 45–64 years.[35] The likelihood of an early death was ten times greater for younger homeless women than for women in the general population.

The State of Housing and Homelessness

According to the Canada Mortgage and Housing Corporation: "Affordable housing costs less than 30% of before-tax household income." Its data show that a significant proportion of Canadian households experience housing affordability issues, and this proportion increased between 1991 and 2006. This situation is especially the case for Canadian renters, a situation associated with low levels of income and wealth.[36]

In addition, the proportion of tenants in Canadian cities spending more than 30 percent of their total income on rent is high (43 percent in Vancouver, 42 percent in Toronto, and 36 percent in Montreal. The proportion spending more than 50 percent — putting them at risk of imminent homelessness — is also strikingly high (22 percent in Vancouver, 20 percent in Toronto, and 18 percent in Montreal). Rental costs have far outpaced income increases among low-income renters in virtually all Canadian urban areas (for Vancouver the discrepancy is 45 percent; for Toronto, 62 percent; Montreal data is not available).[37]

Michael Shapcott of the Wellesley Institute in Toronto points out that profound shifts have occurred in housing policy in Canada since the mid-1980s.[38] From the end of World War II until 1993 the federal government (with some cost-sharing from the provinces) funded about 650,000 housing units for low-income Canadians. Like many provinces, Ontario funded a social housing program from the mid-1980s to 1995.

After the election of a Conservative government in 1984, the federal government began to withdraw its commitment to housing. Within ten years almost $2 billion had been withdrawn from housing programs, and all new social housing had been cancelled. The election of a Liberal government in 1993 led to a 1996 announcement of plans to end all federal government involvement in the provision of affordable housing. More recently the pronounced increase in homelessness in Canada that resulted from these shifts led to growing pressures on the federal government to respond, and in December 1999, it implemented a national homelessness strategy. A key component of this initiative was the Supporting Community Partnerships Initiative (SCPI), which provided $753 million over three years to create innovative transitional housing and services in several cities.

In November 2001 the federal government signed the Affordable Housing Framework Agreement with every province and territory. The federal government agreed to provide $1 billion over five years. Provinces and territories agreed to match the federal dollars. However, Shapcott points out:

- Most provinces are not paying their matching share. The definition of "affordable" has been changed to "average market rents," so the new housing will be rented at existing market rents. However, as many as two-thirds of renters cannot afford average rents, which puts the housing out of the reach of those who need it the most.

- Even if the framework agreement was fully funded, the total number of units would be well short of the amount required to meet the massive and growing need for affordable rental housing.[39]

Recommendations for Improving Housing Security and Reducing Homelessness

Researchers have noted that it is well within the reach of Canadian governments to end the homelessness crisis by increasing their budgetary allocation for housing by 1 percent of total overall spending.

Shapcott notes that in September 2005, the federal, provincial, and territorial housing ministers met in White Point, Nova Scotia and created "principles for a new Canadian Housing Framework." They promised to "accelerate work" on the new housing framework, but "then didn't even schedule another meeting until February 2008, more than two and a half years later." Remarkably, the federal housing minister refused to even attend the meeting, but under significant pressure agreed to meet with his provincial and territorial counterparts two months later. These meetings have led to a collection of agreements being released, but Shapcott argues that these moves do not come close to replacing the massive reductions made to housing programs during the 1990s. He states:

> The One Percent Solution calls for an additional $2 billion in annual federal spending on top of the $2 billion currently being spent. Other recent national housing proposals, including the January 2008 plan from the Federation of Canadian Municipalities, call for a similar scale of response (the FCM target is $3.35 billion).[40]

Even before the onset of the current recession, the possibility of the

One Percent Solution being implemented seemed unlikely — and it seems even less likely now.

Early Childhood Development, Food, and Housing = Better Health

The situation concerning the social determinants of early child development, food security, and housing in Canada is disturbing — and

---

One Percent Solution to the Housing Crisis

In 1998 the Toronto Disaster Relief Committee (TDRC) launched a national campaign called the One Percent Solution. The campaign grew out of an observation by Dr. David Hulchanski, a leading Canadian housing scholar. He noted that in the early 1990s the federal, provincial, territorial, and municipal governments spent about 1 percent of their overall budgets on housing. The TDRC figured that doubling that amount — or adding an additional 1 percent — would create an envelope to fund a comprehensive, national housing strategy.

In its 2000 pre-budget submission to the House of Commons Standing Committee on Finance, the Toronto Disaster Relief Committee joined with the National Housing and Homelessness Network (NHHN) to renew the call for implementation of the One Percent Solution. The enhanced funding envelope, combined with existing housing spending, would allow the federal government to adopt a comprehensive national housing strategy with these key elements:

- supply (increase the number of rental units)
- affordability (ensure the new units are affordable to the households that need the new housing the most)
- supports (programs for those who require special services)
- rehabilitation (funding to maintain housing to a proper standard)
- emergency relief (special support for people who are already homeless)

Source: *The One Percent Solution*, The Toronto Disaster Relief Committee, Toronto, 1998.

we have every reason to believe that the situation has only worsened since the onset of the 2008 recession.

In 1998 the Toronto Disaster Relief Committee declared homelessness a national disaster. Considering the situation of children in Canada and the crisis of food and housing insecurity, additional calls to direct attention to the situation of children, food, and housing insecurity would be timely. Canada is a signatory to numerous United Nations covenants and agreements that call attention to meeting the basic needs of its citizens, but all the evidence indicates that Canada is failing to meet its obligations under these agreements.

Notes

1. M. Friendly. 2009. "Early Childhood Education and Care as a Social Determinant of Health." In D. Raphael (ed.), *Social Determinants Of Health: Canadian Perspectives*. Second edition. Toronto: Canadian Scholars' Press.

2. M. Rioux. 2010. "The Right to Health: Human Rights Approaches to Health." In T. Bryant, D. Raphael, and M. Rioux (eds.), *Staying Alive: Critical Perspectives on Health, Illness, and Health Care*. Second edition. Toronto: Canadian Scholars. Press.

3. C. Hertzman. 2001. "Population Health and Child Development: A View from Canada." In J.A. Auerbach and B. Krimgold (eds.), *Income, Socioeconomic Status, and Health: Exploring the Relationships*. Washington, DC: National Policy Association.

4. C. Hertzman. 1999. "The Biological Embedding of Early Experience and Its Effects on Health in Adulthood." *Annals of the New York Academy of Sciences* 896: 85–95.

5. C. Hertzman and M. Wiens. 1996. "Child Development and Long-Term Outcomes: A Population Health Perspective and Summary of Successful Interventions." *Social Science and Medicine* 43 (7): 1083–95.

6. A. Antonovsky. 1987. *Unraveling the Mystery of Health: How People Manage Stress and Stay Well*. San Francisco: Jossey Bass; J. Lynch, G. Kaplan, and J. Salonen. 1997. "Why Do Poor People Behave Poorly? Variation in Adult Health Behaviours and Psychosocial Characteristics by Stages of the Socioeconomic Lifecourse." *Social Science and Medicine* 44 (6): 809–19.

7. J.D. Willms (ed.). 2002. *Vulnerable Children: Findings from Canada's National*

Longitudinal Survey. Edmonton, AB: University of Alberta Press.

8. J.D. Willms. 2003. "Literacy Proficiency of Youth: Evidence of Converging Socioeconomic Gradients." *International Journal of Educational Research* 39: 247–52.

9. D. Evans, C. Hertzman, and S. Morgan. 2007. "Improving Health Outcomes in Canada." In J. Leonard, C. Ragan, and F. St-Hilaire (eds.), *A Canadian Priorities Agenda: Policy Choices to Improve Economic and Social Well-Being.* Ottawa: Institute for Research on Public Policy.

10. C. Hertzman and C. Power. 2003. "Health and Human Development: Understandings from Life-Course Research." *Developmental Neuropsychology* 24 (2&3): 719–44.

11. Campaign 2000. 2009. *2009 Report Card on Child and Family Poverty In Canada: 1989–2009.* Toronto: Campaign 2000. According to Statistics Canada, the percentage of Canadian children living in these circumstances (pre-tax) was 15 percent in 2007. This figure is virtually unchanged from 1989 when the House of Commons unanimously voted to eliminate child poverty in Canada by the year 2000.

12. Organisation for Economic Co-operation and Development (OECD). 2009. *Growing Unequal: Income Distribution and Poverty in OECD Nations.* Paris: OECD.

13. Innocenti Research Centre. 2008. *The Child Care Transition: A League Table of Early Childhood Education and Care in Economically Advanced Countries. Report Card No. 6.* Florence: Innocenti Research Centre.

14. Newfoundland and Labrador Business Coalition. 2008. *Submission to the 2008 Minimum Wage Review: Impacts on Business.* St. John's: Newfoundland and Labrador Business Coalition.

15. Innocenti Research Centre. 2005. *Child Poverty in Rich Nations, 2005. Report Card No. 6.* Florence: Innocenti Research Centre; Innocenti Research Centre.

16. L. McIntyre and K. Rondeau. 2009. "Food Insecurity in Canada." In D. Raphael (ed.), *Social Determinants of Health: Canadian Perspectives.* Second edition. Toronto: Canadian Scholars Press.

17. L. McIntyre and K. Rondeau. 2009. "Food Insecurity in Canada." In D. Raphael (ed.), *Social Determinants of Health: Canadian Perspectives.* Second edition. Toronto: Canadian Scholars Press.

18. L. McIntyre and K. Rondeau. 2009.

19. Canadian Association of Food Banks. 2009. *Hungercount 2009: A Comprehensive Report on Hunger and Food Bank Use in Canada and Recommendations for Change.* Toronto: CAFB.

20. S.I. Kirkpatrick and V. Tarasuk. 2008. "Food Insecurity Is Associated

with Nutrient Inadequacies among Canadian Adults and Adolescents." *Journal of Nutrition* 138 (3): 604–12.

21. V. Tarasuk. 2009. "Food Insecurity and Health." In D. Raphael (ed.), *Social Determinants of Health: Canadian Perspectives.* Second edition. Toronto: Canadian Scholars' Press: p. 214.

22. V. Tarasuk. 2009. "Food Insecurity and Health." In D. Raphael (ed.), *Social Determinants of Health: Canadian Perspectives.* Second edition. Toronto: Canadian Scholars' Press: p. 214; N. Vozoris and V. Tarasuk. 2003. "Household Food Insufficiency Is Associated with Poorer Health." *Journal of Nutrition* 133: 120–27.

23. V. Tarasuk. 2009. "Food Insecurity and Health." In D. Raphael (ed.), *Social Determinants of Health: Canadian Perspectives.* Second edition. Toronto: Canadian Scholars' Press: p. 218.

24. L. McIntyre and K. Rondeau. 2009. "Food Insecurity in Canada." In D. Raphael (ed.), *Social Determinants of Health: Canadian Perspectives*. Second edition. Toronto: Canadian Scholars Press.

25. L. McIntyre and K. Rondeau. 2009.

26. World Health Organization. 1986. *Ottawa Charter for Health Promotion.* Geneva: World Health Organization.

27. J. Engeland, R. Lewis, S. Ehrlich, and J. Che. 2005. *Evolving Housing Conditions in Canada's Census Metropolitan Areas, 1991–2001.* Ottawa: Statistics Canada and the Canada Mortgage and Housing Corporation.

28. T. Bryant. 2009. "Housing and Health: More than Bricks and Mortar." In D. Raphael (ed.), *Social Determinants of Health: Canadian Perspectives.* Second edition. Toronto: Canadian Scholars' Press.

29. S. Hwang et al. 1999. "Housing and Population Health: A Review of the Literature." Toronto: Centre for Applied Social Research Faculty of Social Work, University of Toronto.

30. A. Savage. 1988. *Warmth in Winter: Evaluation of an Information Pack for Elderly People.* Cardiff: Cardiff University of Wales College of Medicine Research Team for the Care of the Elderly; D. Strachan. 1988. "Damp Housing and Childhood Asthma: Validation of Reporting of Symptoms." *British Medical Journal* 297: 1223–26; S. Platt, C. Martin, S. Hunt, and C. Lewis. 1989. "Damp Housing, Mould Growth and Symptomatic Health State." *British Medical Journal* 298: 1673–78.

31. T. Bryant. 2009. "Housing and Health: More than Bricks and Mortar." In D. Raphael (ed.), *Social Determinants of Health: Canadian Perspectives.* Second edition. Toronto: Canadian Scholars' Press: p. 240.

32. A. Marsh, D. Gordon, C. Pantazis, and P. Heslop. 1999. *Home Sweet Home? The Impact of Poor Housing on Health.* Bristol: Policy Press.

33. D.J. Dedman et al. 2001. "Childhood Housing Conditions and Later Mortality in the Boyd Orr Cohort." *Journal of Epidemiology and Community Health* 55: 10–15.

34. E. Ambrosio, D. Baker, C. Crowe and K. Hardill. 1992. *The Street Health Report: A Study of the Health Status and Barriers to Health Care of Homeless Women and Men in the City of Toronto.* Toronto: Street Health.

35. C. Kushner. 1998. *Better Access, Better Care: A Research Paper on Health Services and Homelessness In Toronto.* Toronto: Toronto Mayor's Homelessness Action Task Force; S. Hwang. 2001. "Homelessness and Health." *Canadian Medical Association Journal* 164 (2): 229–33; A. Cheung and S. Hwang. 2004. "Risk of Death among Homeless Women: A Cohort Study and Review of the Literature." *Canadian Medical Association Journal* 170 (8): 1243–47.

36. Canada Mortgage and Housing Corporation. 2009. "Housing in Canada On-line." <http://data.beyond2020.com/cmhc/HiCODefinitions_EN.html#_Affordable_dwellings_1>; D. Hulchanski. 2001. *A Tale of Two Canadas: Homeowners Getting Richer, Renters Getting Poorer.* Toronto: Centre For Urban and Community Studies, University of Toronto; D. Hulchanski. 2007. *The Three Cities within Toronto: Income Polarization Among Toronto's Neighbourhoods, 1970–2000.* Toronto: Centre for Urban and Community Studies, University of Toronto.

37. Statistics Canada. 2004. *Owner Households and Tenant Households by Major Payments and Gross Rent as a Percentage of 1995 Household Income, 1996 Census, Census Metropolitan Areas.* Ottawa: Statistics Canada; Federation of Canadian Municipalities. 2004. *Income, Shelter and Necessities.* Ottawa: Federation of Canadian Municipalities.

38. M. Shapcott. 2009. "Housing." In D. Raphael (ed.), *Social Determinants of Health: Canadian Perspectives.* Second edition. Toronto: Canadian Scholars' Press.

39. M. Shapcott. 2009. "Housing." In D. Raphael (ed.), *Social Determinants of Health: Canadian Perspectives.* Second edition. Toronto: Canadian Scholars' Press: p. 231.

40. M. Shapcott. 2009. "Housing." In D. Raphael (ed.), *Social Determinants of Health: Canadian Perspectives.* Second edition. Toronto: Canadian Scholars' Press: p. 232.

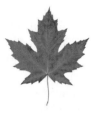

5. SOCIAL EXCLUSION

Aboriginal Status, Race, Gender, and Disability

> The rhetoric of multicultural harmony and embracing diversity that has been a part of Canadian government policy over the past 20 years does not jibe with the reality of increasing inequality between the racialized communities and other Canadians. —Grace-Edward Galabuzi, 2009

In Canada the all too many people are who are most vulnerable to material and social disadvantage — those with low incomes and no-wealth, Aboriginal Canadians, people of colour, recent immigrants, women, and people with disabilities — are undoubtedly those who experience the bitter side of the social determinants of health. But they also have less power than do other Canadians to influence governments and policy-makers. Certain groups of Canadians are denied the opportunity to participate in a wide range of activities that should be readily available to all members of society.[1] That situation and the processes by which it occurs have come to be called "social exclusion." And it is these excluded Canadians whose health is especially at risk.

Defining Social Exclusion

Paul White of the University of Sheffield identifies four key aspects of social exclusion.[2] The first is a denial of participation in civil affairs as a result of legal sanction or other institutional mechanisms. This occurs when laws and regulations prevent non-status residents or migrants from participating in a variety of societal activities. It may also include systemic forms of discrimination based on race, gender, ethnicity, or disability status, among other factors. A relevant example is new Canadians — the case of physicians and nurses comes to mind — not being able to practise their professions due to myriad regulations and procedures that effectively bar their participation. For example, while Ontario garners more than 50 percent of immigrants to Canada, including a large number of physicians who were licensed in their homelands, at the end of the 1990s only twenty-four residency positions were available to internationally trained physicians. If there were a large number of graduates from local medical schools they received the spots, not the new Canadians. Towards the end of the 2000s the number had improved to two hundred spots a year, but there were still many more applicants than spots available.[3]

The second form of social exclusion is the denial of social goods such as health care, education, housing, income security, and language services, and the lack of a means of reducing discrimination. Some marginalized groups — Aboriginal Canadians, people of colour, recent immigrants, women, and people with disabilities — experience lower income than do Canadians of European descent. They are more likely to experience a lack of affordable housing and to find it more difficult to get access to necessary medical services.

The third type of exclusion is called "exclusion from social production," which involves a denial of the opportunity to participate in and contribute to social and cultural activities. Much of this deprivation has to do with the lack of financial resources experienced by specific groups in Canadian society. "Economic exclusion" is the fourth type, and it denotes cases in which individuals cannot get access to economic resources and opportunities such as participation in paid work. Evidence shows systematic differences in unemployment levels, employment insecurity, and training opportunities among non-disabled Canadians of European descent and members of the other groups. Social exclusion has a huge impact on many important social determinants of health.

As Janie Percy-Smith of Leeds Metropolitan University tells us, the incidence and experience of social exclusion must be examined within the local situation.[4] Particular aspects of local places, populations, and governmental decisions shape whether citizens are able to participate in activities that are expected to be open to all citizens of a nation. Consider the situation of your local jurisdiction and the extent to which vulnerable groups are systematically excluded from day-to-day participation. Until recently Ontario offered virtually no opportunity for foreign-trained physicians to receive certification in their profession.

These aspects are themselves embedded within a national context that has particular economic and political approaches to the provision of citizen security and the distribution of resources. Clearly, Canada has been lagging in providing such security, creating a skewed distribution of resources. Related to this is the manner in which a nation responds to economic globalization. Does a nation ensure that the effects of globalization will not have a negative impact on the population in general and the most vulnerable in particular? Many European Union nations, for example, provide extensive supports for people who experience unemployment as a result of globalization. These supports include replacement benefits close to their usual earnings as well as retraining opportunities.

The opposite approach occurs when a government hesitates to intervene to mitigate the adverse effects of globalization. That is the case in Canada where many unemployed citizens are unable to get access to unemployment benefits or retraining opportunities. Finally, all of this takes place against the ongoing international restructuring of economic markets, the process that we have come to know as economic globalization.

Evidence indicates that Canadian governments at all levels have done little to mitigate the harmful effects of globalization. Indeed, public policy professor Grace-Edward Galabuzi of Ryerson University argues that processes of social exclusion — especially among the most vulnerable groups — have been accelerated by the restructuring of Canada's economy and labour market to be consistent with the neo-liberal visions of society.[5] This vision includes increasing the dominance of the corporate sector and "the market," allowing these entities — rather than the government in the form of various public policies — to be the prime judges of how resources are distributed amongst Canadians. This approach has resulted in the growing income and wealth inequality and persistence of high levels of poverty in Canada.

Canada's response to the demands of globalization has been increased temporary and insecure employment, stagnating wages, and the limiting of governmental spending on benefits, programs, and services. The neo-liberal restructuring of the economy, therefore, has a large impact on the social determinants of health, especially in the cases of the most vulnerable people. Social exclusion is both the process and result of this restructuring of the economy.

Aboriginal Peoples and Health

The health of Aboriginal peoples in Canada — the First Nations, Dene, Métis, and Inuit — and elsewhere is inextricably tied up with their history of colonization.[6] In Canada this history has taken the form of legislation such as the *Indian Act* of 1876, disregard for the land claims of Métis peoples, relocation of Inuit communities, and the establishment of residential schools. Dislocations removed many Aboriginal people from their lands and undermined their economies and livelihoods. The result has been manifested in the social determinants of health, leading to adverse health outcomes.

In 2006 the Aboriginal peoples numbered 1.2 million and con-stituted about 3.8 percent of the Canadian population. Sociologist Martin Cooke of the University of Waterloo and his colleagues show the gap in life expectancy between Aboriginal and non-Aboriginal Canadians in 2001 to be almost six years.[7] Another gap comes in the form of income. As physician and research scientist Janet Smylie points out, in 2001 the average income of Aboriginal men and women was $21,958 and $16,529 respectively, which represented 58 percent of the average income of non-Aboriginal men and 72 percent of the average income of non-Aboriginal women.[8] For Aboriginal Canadians living on reserves, their respective figures as a percent-age of non-Aboriginal incomes were, for men, 40 percent, and for women, 61 percent. For those living off-reserve the figures were somewhat better but still well below the incomes of non-Aboriginal Canadians. Similarly, in 2001, 26 percent of Aboriginal households had incomes below the low-income cut-offs, in contrast to the 12 percent figures for households that were not Aboriginal.

In 2001 the Aboriginal Canadian unemployment rate was 14 percent, which was double the rate of non-Aboriginal households. For First Nations Canadians living on-reserve the figure was 28 percent, which was twice the rate for Aboriginals living off-reserve. Education levels also differ widely between Aboriginal and other Canadians.

Table 5-1. Educational Attainment Levels: Aboriginal vs. Non-Aboriginal Canadians, 2001

High School Attainment					
	First Nation On-Reserve	First Nation Off-Reserve	Inuit	Métis	Non-Aboriginal
Men	40%	56%	43%	65%	71%
Women	43%	57%	43%	63%	70%

Adapted from: J. Smyley, "The Health of Aboriginal People," in D. Raphael (ed.), *Social Determinants of Health: Canadian Perspectives,* second edition, Toronto: Canadian Scholars' Press, 2009.

Key Elements of the Colonization of Aboriginal People in Canada

The *Indian Act*

"The first *Indian Act* of 1876 reflects governmental policies of assimilation of Aboriginal populations in Canada and appropriation of Aboriginal lands.... The Constitution Act of 1867 and subsequent *Indian Acts* legalized the removal of First Nations communities, which had signed treaties, from their homelands to 'reserve lands' that were controlled by the Government of Canada on behalf of 'Indians.' The *Indian Acts* of 1876, 1880, and 1884 later outlawed First Nations ceremonies such as the sundance and potlatch and gave the Indian agent authority over the foods, goods, and travel available to on-reserve First Nations peoples. These policies also supported the abduction of Aboriginal children to residential schools, where language and culture were actively suppressed."

Disregard of Métis Land Claims

"In 1869, the Hudson Bay Company transferred its lands in Canada's Northwest and authority for these lands to the Government of Canada.... At the time of the transfer, First Nations and Métis were by far the biggest populations living in these areas.... This transfer did not include any provision for the First Nations and Métis peoples who were living on these lands, and social unrest was therefore a predictable outcome.... The disruption of Métis families and communities resulting from federal governmental disregard for and appropriation of their lands has had a long-standing impact on Métis.... Prior to the Hudson Bay land transfer in Manitoba and the uprising in Batoche, many Métis families on the Prairies were economically prospering. Following these events, Métis struggled economically and commonly faced racial prejudice from European settlers, which, in turn, limited job prospects."

Relocation of Inuit Communities

"During and after the Second World War, the federal government had a policy of 'encouraging' Inuit to relocate into permanent villages in areas selected by the government.... One of the first relocation attempts occurred in 1934. Twenty-two Inuit from Kinngait (Cape Dorset), 18 from Mittimatalk/Tununiq (Pond Inlet), and 12 from Pangnirtuuq (Pangnirtung) were transported to Dundas Harbour. During the 1950s and 1960s, many more Inuit families were moved from their traditional lands to permanent settlements. The hunting conditions of the new sites were usually suboptimal, interfering with traditional food supply. In addition to food insecurity, unemployment, and housing issues, the move to permanent settlements was accompanied by outbreaks of tuberculosis. By 1964, more than 70 percent of Keewatin Inuit had been in TB sanatoria."

Source: J. Smylie, "The Health of Aboriginal People," in D. Raphael (ed.), *Social Determinants of Health: Canadian Perspectives,* second edition, Toronto: Canadian Scholars' Press, 2009.

The level of food insecurity is strikingly high. Aboriginal Canadians living off-reserve were four times more likely to experience food insecurity than were non-Aboriginal Canadians. Some 33 percent of off-reserve Aboriginal households experienced moderate or severe food insecurity in 2004 as compared to 8.8 percent of non-Aboriginal households. Some 14 percent of Aboriginal households experienced severe food insecurity as compared to 2.7 percent of non-Aboriginal households.

On-reserve food is equally insecure. In the Cree community of Fort Severn, Ontario, for example, two-thirds of households experienced food insecurity in 2002. A 1997 study in the northern communities of Repulse Bay and Pond Inlet found about 50 percent of each community's families reported not having enough to eat in the previous thirty days.[9] Aboriginal peoples are also four times more likely to be living in crowded housing. Some 38 percent of Inuit in Innuit Nunatt live in crowded housing, as compared to 11 percent of Aboriginal Canadians and 3 percent of the non-Aboriginal population.

The life expectancies of Aboriginal peoples are five to fourteen years less than that of the Canadian population, with Inuit men and women showing the shortest lives.[10] Among Aboriginal Canadians infant mortality rates — that is, children dying before their first year — are one and a half to four times greater than the overall Canadian rate.

The rates of numerous infectious and chronic diseases are also much higher in the Aboriginal population. Suicide rates are five to six times higher than in the non-Aboriginal Canadian population and Aboriginal peoples have high rates of major depression (18 percent), problems with alcohol (27 percent), and experience of sexual abuse during childhood (34 percent).

Policy Solutions

The United Nations Declaration of the Rights of Indigenous Peoples, approved by the U.N. General Assembly in 2007, identifies numerous areas in which national governments could work to improve the situation of Aboriginal peoples. The Declaration includes articles concerned with improving economic and social conditions, the right to attain the highest levels of health, and the right to protect and conserve their environments. Sadly, Canada was one of the few nations to vote against its adoption.

The 1996 Royal Commission on Aboriginal Peoples (RCAP) included a number of policy recommendations:

- legislation, including a new Royal Proclamation stating Canada's commitment to a new relationship and companion legislation setting out a treaty process and recognition of Aboriginal nations and governments;
- recognition of an Aboriginal order of government, subject to the Charter of Rights and Freedoms, with authority over matters related to the good government and welfare of Aboriginal peoples and their territories;

First Five Articles of the United Nations Declaration on the Rights of Indigenous Peoples

Article 1
Indigenous peoples have the right to the full enjoyment, as a collective or as individuals, of all human rights and fundamental freedoms as recognized in the Charter of the United Nations, the Universal Declaration of Human Rights and international human rights law.

Article 2
Indigenous peoples and individuals are free and equal to all other peoples and individuals and have the right to be free from any kind of discrimination, in the exercise of their rights, in particular that based on their indigenous origin or identity.

Article 3
Indigenous peoples have the right to self-determination. By virtue of that right they freely determine their political status and freely pursue their economic, social and cultural development.

Article 4
Indigenous peoples, in exercising their right to self-determination, have the right to autonomy or self-government in matters relating to their internal and local affairs, as well as ways and means for financing their autonomous functions.

Article 5
Indigenous peoples have the right to maintain and strengthen their distinct political, legal, economic, social and cultural institutions, while retaining their right to participate fully, if they so choose, in the political, economic, social and cultural life of the State.

Source: United Nations, 2007 <http://www2.ohchr.org/english/issues/indigenous/declaration.htm>.

- replacement of the federal Department of Indian Affairs with two departments, one to implement the new relationship with Aboriginal nations and one to provide services for non-self-governing communities;
- creation of an Aboriginal Parliament;
- Expansion of the Aboriginal land and resource base;
- recognition of Métis self-government, provision of a land base, and recognition of Métis rights to hunt and fish on Crown land;
- initiatives to address social, education, health, and housing needs, including the training of ten thousand health professionals over a ten-year period, the establishment of an Aboriginal peoples' university, and recognition of Aboriginal nations' authority over child welfare. [11]

Yet, as Smylie points out, the current state of inaction on these recommendations is striking. In the decade or so after the release of the RCAP report, she saw only "some slow progress in the area of Aboriginal-controlled health services, as well as the identification of Aboriginal health human resources." To Canada's great shame, she also notes, "the Canadian government's lack of implementation of the RCAP recommendations has been extensively criticized by national and international human rights bodies, including the Canadian Human Rights Commission, the United Nations Human Rights Committee, and the United Nations Committee on Economic, Social, and Cultural Rights."[12]

New Canadians, People of Colour, and Health

Immigration during the 1990s accounted for more than half of the increases in the Canadian population and 70 percent of the increases in the number of people in the workplace. By 2011 immigration will account for all of the net growth in the labour force.[13] Since the 1960s over three-quarters of the immigrants to Canada have come from the global South or developing nations; the majority of them are "racialized" immigrants (what were once called "visible minorities"). One-third of the members of racialized groups in Canada are Canadian-born; the other two-thirds are immigrants.

Members of racialized groups in Canada experience a whole range of difficult living circumstances that undermine their general well-being and health. The problematic income situation of new Canadians is common across virtually all immigrant groups to Canada (see Table 5-2). The average income for all of these groups tends to be well below that of Canadian earners in general. Unemployment rates are higher (6.7 percent for Canadian-born workers, 7.9 percent for all immigrants, and 12.1 percent for recent immigrants). Labour force participation is lower: 80.3 percent for

Table 5-2. Average Income (All Sources) by Selected Racialized Community, 2001

	Men	Women	Total
All Canadian earners	36,800	22,885	29,769
African community	27,864	19,639	23,787
Arab community	32,336	19,264	26,519
Caribbean community	29,840	22,842	25,959
Chinese community	29,322	20,974	25,018
Filipino community	27,612	22,532	24,563
Jamaican community	30,087	23,575	26,412
Haitian community	21,595	18,338	19,782
Japanese community	43,644	24,556	33,178
Korean community	23,370	16,919	20,065
Latin American community	27,257	17,930	22,463
South Asian community	31,396	19,511	25,629
Vietnamese community	27,849	18,560	23,190
West Asian community	28,719	18,014	23,841

Source: Statistics Canada, *2001 Census of Canada: 2001 Census Analysis Series — The Changing Profile of Canada's Labour Force*, Catalogue no. 96F0030XIE2001009, February 2003, Ottawa: Statistics Canada. Taken from G.E. Galabuzi, "Social Exclusion," in D. Raphael (ed.), *Social Determinants of Health: Canadian Perspectives*, second edition, Toronto: Canadian Scholars' Press, 2009.

Canadian-born workers, 75.6 percent for all immigrants, and 65.8 percent for recent immigrants.

New immigrants of colour — people who have recently arrived in Canada — show particularly pronounced increases in poverty. Sociologist Michael Ornstein of York University provides dramatic evidence of the adverse living conditions experienced by new immigrants to Canada.[14] He compares the average income of a range of groups (Aboriginal, Arab and West Asian, South Asian, East Asian, African, Caribbean, and South and Central American) to the average income of residents of European descent. In 1971 for women, the average income of these groups was close to the European descent group. Indeed, the incomes of South Asian and West Asian women were higher than those of the European descent average. But over the period of 1970 to 2000 the average income of all of these groups declined relative to the European descent group such that their average incomes were at 70 percent to 80 percent of the European descent group.

For men, the results were equally dramatic. In 1970 the income of men in these groups was already falling behind the incomes of those of European descent, averaging about 75 percent to 85 percent of their levels. The one exception was for Asian and West Asian men, whose incomes were 10 percent higher than those of men of European descent. But by 2000, even the average incomes of Asian and West Asian men had declined to 75 percent of European descent men. The rest of the groups' averages were from 60 percent to 75 percent of men of European descent.

While the average poverty rates for those of European descent were slightly over 10 percent, the figures for other groups were strikingly high: Aboriginal (20 percent); Arab and West Asian (30 percent); South Asian (20 percent); East Asian (20 percent); African (39 percent); Caribbean (22 percent); and South and Central American (20 percent). Like the figures for average income, poverty rates show a striking increase for each group from the period of 1970 to 2000. These patterns are similar for the rest of Canada.[15]

In the past, large-scale surveys did not find — outside of studies of Aboriginal Peoples — significant health differences between racial groups in Canada. Much of this was probably due to the "healthy immigrant effect," whereby immigrants — many of them persons of colour — showed superior health status to non-Aboriginal people born in Canada.[16]

However, a 2005 study from the National Population Health Survey provides compelling evidence that the health of non-European immigrants has deteriorated over time as compared to Canadian-born non-Aboriginal residents and European immigrants. Compared to the Canadian-born population, recent non-European immigrants (less than ten years in Canada) were twice as likely to report deterioration in health from 1993 to 2003. Long-term non-European immigrants were also more likely to report such deterioration, though recent or long-term European immigrants did not. Of

The Lived Experience of Social Exclusion

"The kids… feel isolated and people look down on them because they are living here and they join schools where all the schoolmates are immigrants. So they will never… they will always consider themselves second degree citizens and even outside the school they will always go home because the neighbourhood is dangerous and we're afraid they will get addicted or be involved in other crimes. So they are staying home all the time…"

"Well ma'am you know the neighbourhood you live in. It's either junkies, or addicts, or homeless that live in that neighbourhood."

"When they know that we come from Regent Park, people think that we are bad."

Source: H. Smith and D. Ley, "The Immigrant Experience of Poverty in Toronto: Neighbourhoods of Concentrated Disadvantage," presentation at the Ninth National Metropolis Conference, Toronto, March 1–4, 2007.

importance was the finding that non-European immigrants were 50 percent more likely to become frequent visitors to doctors than were the Canadian-born population.[17]

A number of social determinants of health were related to this trend: income inadequacy, lower levels of education, and a lack of support from others. More recent studies indicate that recent immigrants of colour are coming to experience greater incidences of mental health problems and housing and food insecurity than are Canadians of European descent.[18] The pattern of increasing economic and racial concentration in Canadian urban areas is another cause for concern. In the United States a concentration of economically disadvantaged racialized groups has been associated with adverse health outcomes.[19]

Policy Solutions

In the past, immigrants to Canada would gradually reach income and employment levels comparable to the Canadian-born, but this is no longer happening. Statistics Canada has documented differences in income and employment status of recent and earlier immigrants to Canada.[20] In recent years, increases in low-income status are found among immigrants in all education and age groups, including the university-educated. Given that 75 percent of recent immigrants are members of racialized groups, it would appear that racism and discrimination are responsible for these diminishing returns.

What we need, among other things, is the provision of opportunities for foreign-trained professionals to practise their professions in Canada. We need strong enforcement of anti-discrimination laws. Given that people of colour are especially vulnerable to difficult living circumstances, which have an undoubted impact on the social determinants of health, we especially need our governments at all levels to take an active role in addressing these issues.

Women and Health

Women in Canada, more so than men, are particularly subject to social determinants that have a negative effect on their health. Much of this has to do with the responsibility that women traditionally have had for raising children and caring for the health needs of families.[21] Women are less likely to be working full-time and less likely to be eligible for unemployment benefits. Women are more likely to be employed in lower-paying occupations and more likely to experience discrimination in the workplace. In addition, the public policy decisions associated with economic and social security — such as the failure to raise minimum wages or social assistance benefits, the reduction of access to public health services, limitations on the availability of affordable housing or government-supported quality child care, and the introduction of restrictive workfare requirements — disproportionately hurt women more than men.

Because they tend to work part-time, women earn less than men do.[22] They also earn less than men, regardless of occupation. In 2001 women earned about two-thirds of the income of men. Among Canadians working in management, for example, women earn on average $956 a week compared to $1,261 earned by men. Even in occupations dominated by women, such as clerical jobs, women earn less than men ($518 a week compared to $605 a week). The earnings gap represents a number of issues. Women work fewer hours than men, but their hourly wages are also only 80 percent of the wages of men. Even when women work full-time, their earnings equal only 72 percent of that earned by men. Jobs that are dominated by men tend to pay more; even when women work in these fields, they tend to get paid less.

As a 2001 study by Statistics Canada found, when controls for factors such as work experience and job-related responsibilities are applied, gender differences in wages between men and women remain. The report stated, "despite the long list of productivity-related factors, a substantial portion of the gender gap cannot be explained by traditional measures of education and experience. "[23] Indeed, Ann Curry-Stevens points out:

> Despite popular opinion that women have achieved equality with men, women's incomes remain a stubborn 62 percent lower than men ($24,400 instead of $39,300 for total income in 2003). At first glance, one might think that this is a function of choice and that women might work fewer hours to accumulate this income. But when we compare income levels of women who work full-time to those of men who work full-time, the earnings remain inequitable. While there is a significant improvement, female workers still earn only 71 percent of male earnings.[24]

A predominant reason for why women work fewer hours than men is the lack of affordable and quality day care, which forces family responsibilities onto women. Women are usually responsible for dealing with the burden of reconciling work and family. The problem of balancing employment and family contributes to family stress in general and to women's stress in particular. Affordable and high-quality child care is an important means not only of enabling women to participate in the employment workplace as equals to men but also of promoting women's health and well-being.

Women do seem to have a health advantage when it comes to outliving men. As Ann Pedersen of the Centre for Excellence in Women's Health and her colleagues point out, Canadian women have a life expectancy of 79.0 years compared to 76.3 for men.[25] But this apparent health advantage is less impressive when we take sickness and the use of health services into account. Women report more episodes of long-term disability and chronic conditions than men do. The higher mortality rate and lower life expectancy of men compared to women have been misinterpreted to mean that women enjoy superior health. This interpretation completely ignores the higher prevalence of chronic conditions in women, particularly in later life. Moreover, women's health status in terms of life expectancy may be converging with that of men's: the data suggest a narrowing of the gender gap in longevity in industrialized countries, most of it due to improvements in men's life expectancy.[26] Just as women's life expectancy increased dramatically in the middle of the twentieth century as a result of reductions in maternal mortality, the current pattern of life expectancy observed between women and men may not hold in the future.

Policy Solutions

Governments, health authorities, non-governmental organizations, and advocacy groups have outlined various strategies to address women's health issues. Yet these solutions usually focus on aspects of health care and health outcomes such as reproductive health, screening for various forms of cancer, and appropriate prescribing of medications. They tend not to address the social and economic structures that shape women's (and men's) health:

> Action on these more deeply embedded elements of the social structure may require action far beyond the health sector. Moreover, such strategies need to be developed with an awareness of women's lives so that women are truly able to benefit from the initiative. Financial support for caregiving, for example, is currently part of the Employment Insurance scheme in Canada. Unfortunately, access to this program is limited to people who work full-time and therefore many of the people who need this assistance the most—women—are unable to access the program because they do not qualify.[27]

Many of the recommendations provided in the other cases discussed here are also pertinent to the case of women. These suggestions include the provision of living wages and adequate social assistance benefits, affordable housing and child care, and adjustments to make it easier to qualify for employment insurance. Women especially benefit when they are employed in unionized workplaces. Making it easier to organize workplaces would go a long way to improve the situation of women in Canada. Finally, ensuring pay equity and combating discrimination in the workplace are also important means of overcoming the negative results of the social determinants of health in the case of women.

People with Disabilities

Too often disability is seen in medical rather than societal terms. While disability is clearly related to physical and mental functions, the primary issue is whether society is willing to provide the supports and opportunities that are necessary if people with disabilities are to participate fully in Canadian life. The problems that people with disabilities experience have more to do with society's response to their disabilities than with the disabilities themselves.

Canada's public policy responses to the challenges that people with disabilities face generally lag behind those of other wealthy developed nations. People with disabilities are less likely to be employed: over 40 percent of Canadians with disabilities are not in the labour force. When they are employed, they earn less than people without disabilities do. In 2001 the average earnings of the 43 percent of employed people with disabilities were $32,385; the average earnings of the 78.4 percent of employed people without a disability were $38,677.[28]

Those who are not in the workforce are usually forced to rely upon social assistance benefits, which are very low in Canada. In most cities the payments do not bring individuals even close to the poverty lines. Canada is one of the most frugal nations (eighteenth of twenty-three OECD nations) in its allocation of benefits to people with disabilities.[29]

The Canadian Council on Social Development reports that much of the distress has to do with the workplace being either unable or unwilling to accommodate the needs of persons with disabilities: "Among unemployed persons with disabilities, 56% say they require some type of work aid or job modification, with job redesign (required by 42%) and modified work hours (35%) being the most commonly cited." Ironically, as the Council points out, many of the required modifications are rather minor. The Council summarizes findings from a report issued by the Alberta Abilities Foundation:

> While the requirement for workplace accommodations is fairly high, these accommodations are usually not terribly costly.... [The] annual workplace accommodation costs are under $1,500 for almost all workers who have a disability... for just over half of those requiring some type of accommodation, the estimated cost would be less than $500 per person per year; for one-third, the cost would be $500 to $1,500 per year; and for 16%, the cost was estimated at over $1,500. These costs are probably much lower than many employers realize. For many persons with disabilities, an employer's reluctance to provide accommodation on the job can be extremely disheartening and frustrating: "Employers are still ignorant about what it takes to hire and accommodate a person with a disability."[30]

Policy Solutions

The Council of Canadians with Disabilities and the Canadian Association for Community Living outline various short-term and long-term strategies to improve the situation of Canadians with disabilities.[31] Their short-term strategies call for the federal government to take a number of steps.

> 1. Commit to a Framework for Investment in Disability Supports that will assist individuals to meet the costs of disability-related supports; support family/informal

caregivers; and enable community capacity to provide supports and inclusion.

2. Implement recommendations to Ministers of Finance and Revenue in Disability Tax Fairness.

3. Make a "downpayment" on a transfer to enhance the supply of disability supports, and commit to a national program for wider investments in disability supports.

4. Commit to a "disability dimension" in new initiatives, including Caregivers, Childcare, Cities and Communities, and the Gas Tax Rebate. The federal government commitment to "universal inclusion" should be made in infrastructure initiatives for cities and communities, including the Gas Tax Rebate, to enhance accessible transportation and other services.

5. Commit to a study of poverty and disability as a foundation for exploring an expanded role for the federal government in addressing income needs.

6. Engage the disability community and provincial/territorial governments in developing the agenda by providing the disability community with the resources necessary to effectively work on this project, and by establishing a new high-level Technical Advisory Group to advise the federal government on the agenda.

The long-term strategies are to:

1. explore a further role for the federal government in addressing poverty, by meeting individual costs of disability through an expenditure program, perhaps modelled after the National Child Benefit.

2. integrate the Caregiver Agenda into a Framework for Investment in Disability Supports.

Numerous organizations have also suggested raising benefit

levels for persons with disabilities who are unable to work. As it now stands, Canada has one of the least developed approaches towards assisting persons with disabilities.

Social Inclusion = Better Health

Through the tendencies of social exclusion, certain groups of people are denied the opportunity to participate in civil society. They are denied an acceptable supply of goods or services, essentially unable to contribute to society, and unable to acquire the normal commodities expected of citizens. All of these elements occur in tandem with the experience of material and social deprivation associated with the social determinants of health. These experiences have strong effects upon health.

Social exclusion happens to people as a result of governmental policy and socio-economic structures of racism, sexism, and ableism rather than as a result of the characteristics of individuals. Once again, what all of these groups share in common is a relative lack of power to influence public policy. In essence, it is changing this lack of socio-political power that will do as much for the health of Canadians as all the medical research and health-care improvements that occupy so much public debate and political activity.

Notes

1. G.E. Galabuzi. 2009. "Social Exclusion." In D. Raphael (ed.), *Social Determinants of Health: Canadian Perspectives.* Second edition. Toronto: Canadian Scholars' Press.

2. P. White. 1998. "Ideologies, Social Exclusion and Spatial Segregation in Paris." In S. Mursterd and W. Ostendorf (eds.), *Urban Degradation and the Welfare State: Inequality and Exclusion in Western Cities.* London, UK: Routledge.

3. T. Wojtasiewicz. 2008. "Easing Barriers for Newcomer Physicians." *Canadian Newcomer Magazine* 20 (4).

4. J. Percy-Smith (ed.). 2000. *Policy Responses to Social Exclusion: Towards Inclusion?* Buckingham, UK: Open University Press.

5. G.E. Galabuzi. 2009. "Social Exclusion." In D. Raphael (ed.), *Social Determinants of Health: Canadian Perspectives.* Second edition. Toronto: Canadian Scholars' Press.

6. J. Smylie. 2009. "The Health of Aboriginal People." In D. Raphael (ed.), *Social Determinants of Health: Canadian Perspectives.* Second edition. Toronto: Canadian Scholars' Press. The content on Aboriginal health in Canada is adapted from this source.

7. M. Cooke et al. 2007. "Indigenous Well-being in Four Countries: An Application of the UNDP's Human Development Index to Indigenous Peoples in Australia, Canada, New Zealand, and the United States." *BMC International Health and Human Rights* 7: 9.

8. J. Smylie. 2009. "The Health of Aboriginal People." In D. Raphael (ed.), *Social Determinants of Health: Canadian Perspectives.* Second edition. Toronto: Canadian Scholars' Press.

9. J. Lawn and D. Harvey. 2001. *Change in Food Security and Nutrition in Two Inuit Communities, 1992 to 1997.* Ottawa: Indian and Northern Affairs Canada.

10. J. Smylie. 2009. "The Health of Aboriginal People." In D. Raphael (ed.), *Social Determinants of Health: Canadian Perspectives.* Second edition. Toronto: Canadian Scholars' Press.

11. Royal Commission on Aboriginal Peoples. 1996. *Report of the Royal Commission on Aboriginal Peoples.* Ottawa: Indian and Northern Affairs.

12. J. Smylie. 2009. "The Health of Aboriginal People." In D. Raphael (ed.), *Social Determinants of Health: Canadian Perspectives.* Second edition. Toronto: Canadian Scholars' Press.

13. G.E. Galabuzi. 2009. "Social Exclusion." In D. Raphael (ed.), *Social Determinants of Health: Canadian Perspectives.* Second edition. Toronto: Canadian Scholars' Press.

14. M. Ornstein. 2006. *Ethno-Racial Groups in Toronto, 1971–2001: A Demographic and Social-economic Profile.* Toronto: City of Toronto.

15. G.E. Galabuzi. 2005. *Canada's Economic Apartheid: The Social Exclusion of Racialized Groups in the New Century.* Toronto: Canadian Scholars Press.

16. J. McMullin. 2009. *Understanding Social Inequality: Intersections of Class, Age, Gender, Ethnicity and Race in Canada.* Second edition. Toronto: Oxford University Press; I. Hyman. 2001. *Immigration and Health.* Retrieved July 2002 from <http://www.hc-sc.gc.ca/iacb-dgiac/arad-draa/english/rmdd/wpapers/Immigration.pdf>.

17. E. Ng, R. Wilkins, F. Gendron, and J.M. Berthelot. 2005. *Healthy Today,*

Healthy Tomorrow? Findings from the National Population Health Survey. Ottawa: Statistics Canada.

18. Colour of Poverty. 2009. *Fact Sheets from the Colour of Poverty Project* <http://cop.openconcept.ca>; M. Wallis and S. Kwok (eds.). 2008. *Daily Struggles: The Deepening Racialization and Feminization of Poverty in Canada.* Toronto: Canadian Scholars' Press.

19. N. Ross, K. Nobrega, and J. Dunn. 2001. "Income Segregation, Income Inequality and Mortality in North American Metropolitan Areas." *GeoJournal* 53 (2): 117–24.

20. G. Picot. 2004. *The Deteriorating Economic Welfare of Immigrants and Possible Causes.* Ottawa: Statistics Canada.

21. P. Armstrong. 2009. "Public Policy, Gender, and Health." In D. Raphael (ed.), *Social Determinants of Health: Canadian Perspectives.* Second edition. Toronto: Canadian Scholars' Press.

22. A. Jackson. 2010. *Work and Labour in Canada: Critical Issues.* Second edition. Toronto: Canadian Scholars' Press.

23. M. Drolet. 2001. *The Persistent Gap: New Evidence on the Canadian Gender Wage Gap.* Ottawa: Analytic Studies Branch, Statistics Canada.

24. A. Curry-Stevens. 2009. "When Economic Growth Doesn't Trickle Down: The Wage Dimensions of Income Polarization," In D. Raphael (ed.), *Social Determinants of Health: Canadian Perspectives.* Second edition. Toronto: Canadian Scholars' Press.

25. A. Pederson, D. Raphael, and E. Johnson. 2010. "Gender, Race, and Health Inequalities." In T. Bryant, D. Raphael, and M. Rioux (eds.), *Staying Alive: Critical Perspectives on Health, Illness, and Health Care.* Second edition. Toronto: Canadian Scholars' Press.

26. M. DesMeules, L. Turner, and R. Cho. 2003. "Morbidity Experiences and Disability among Canadian Women." In M. DesMeules et al. (eds.), *Women's Health Surveillance Report: A Multi-dimensional Look at the Health of Canadian Women.* Ottawa: Health Canada, Canadian Population Health Initiative; M.T. Ruiz and L.M. Verbrugge. 1997. "A Two-Way View of Gender Bias in Medicine." *Journal of Epidemiology and Community Health* 51: 106–109; F. Trovato and N.M. Lalu. 1996. "Narrowing Sex Differentials in Life Expectancy in the Industrialized World: Early 1970s to Early 1990s." *Social Biology* 43 (1–2): 20–37.

27. A. Pederson, D. Raphael, and E. Johnson. 2010. "Gender, Race, and Health Inequalities." In T. Bryant, D. Raphael, and M. Rioux (eds.), *Staying Alive: Critical Perspectives on Health, Illness, and Health Care.* Second

edition. Toronto: Canadian Scholars' Press.

28. A. Jackson. 2010. *Work and Labour in Canada: Critical Issues*. Second edition. Toronto: Canadian Scholars' Press.

29. Organisation for Economic Co-operation and Development (OECD). 2009. *Social Expenditure Database*, Available at <http://stats.oecd.org/wbos/default.aspx?datasetcode=SOCX_AGG>.

30. Canadian Council on Social Development. 2005. *Employment and Persons with Disabilities in Canada*. Ottawa: CCSD. The quotation "Employers are still ignorant..." is from Canadian Abilities Foundation. 2004. "Neglected or Hidden." Toronto: p. 9.

31. Council of Canadians with Disabilities. 2005. "A Call to Combat Poverty and Exclusion of Canadians with Disabilities by Investing in Disability Supports." Ottawa: Council of Canadians with Disabilities.

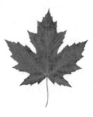

6. PUBLIC POLICY AND THE SOCIAL DETERMINANTS OF HEALTH

Policies shape how money, power and material resources flow through society and therefore affect the determinants of health. Advocating healthy public policies is the most important strategy we can use to act on the determinants of health. — Canadian Public Health Association, "Action Statement for Health Promotion in Canada," 1996

In its 2008 final report, *Closing the Gap in a Generation: Health Equity through Action on the Social Determinants of Health*, the World Health Organization's Commission on Social Determinants of Health sagely noted that the "unequal distribution of health-damaging experiences is not in any sense a 'natural' phenomenon." Rather, it stated, the prevailing conditions are "the result of a toxic combination of poor social policies and programmes, unfair economic arrangements, and bad politics."[1]

In other words, it is an issue that governments not only have helped to create, but also can do something about; and experience in Canada and abroad shows that governments and policy-makers indeed have the ability to shape public policies that will support and encourage health, not damage it. The specific policies that are necessary to achieve this goal have been well documented, and in some cases and countries they have been put into effective practice. Where the policies have been implemented they have resulted in a better quality of life based on a more equitable distribution of the resources that in turn determine the makeup of the social determinants of health — and thus lead to better conditions of health for the population as a whole.

Given that Canada has consistently failed to implement such policies, we need again to consider the economic, political, and ideological forces that prevent the appropriate actions from being taken. One of the problems in this regard is that within the political economy of Canada — that is, the operation of the country's political and economic systems — the marketplace, rather than the government through its laws and regulations, is the dominant institution shaping the structures and conditions that underpin the social determinants of health. The governmental policy-making associated with this form of political economy is generally inconsistent with a perspective that places its priorities, as the World Health Organization puts it, on the "pathways through which social conditions translate into health impacts."[2] To overcome these problems, we must find the means to provide a more reasonable balance between the marketplace and the other sectors of Canadian society whose voices have less influence upon governments and policy-makers.

Shaping a Context for Public Policy

Public policy is a course of action or inaction taken by public authorities — usually governments — to address a given problem or set of problems. These activities are first of all anchored in a set of values and beliefs that shapes whether a situation will even be perceived as being a public — rather than an individual — problem. Then, if it is so perceived, the next step is to define what the appropriate government response should be to address the associated issue.

Numerous examples exist of issues that may or may not be seen as public problems worthy of public policy solutions. Take child care, for example. The importance of families having access to regulated, high-quality, and affordable child care has been fully documented in wealthy developed nations. High-quality child care supports child development, allows women to enter the workforce on equal terms with men, and provides numerous other benefits to the society as a whole, such as providing a well-educated workforce that can both adjust to changes in the workplace and benefit from employment retraining if necessary.[3]

Even so, in many countries, including Canada, the lack of high-quality affordable child care is not universally perceived as a public problem worthy of a public policy solution. It is seen as such in the Scandinavian nations and in many continental European nations, where public policy is influenced by values of promoting gender equity and societal cohesion. This is apparently not the case in Canada, which still lacks the structures to ensure access to high quality affordable public child care.

The role that values play in setting public policy is also starkly apparent when we consider issues related to employment security and working conditions, wages and benefits, and food and housing insecurity. Most European Union nations have labour legislation and regulations that provide employment security and require that benefits and retraining opportunities are provided to both full-time and part-time workers. National commissions ensure that levels of wages and benefits allow citizens to avoid both material and social deprivation and housing and food insecurity. These nations — both social-democratic and continental European — develop public policies that aim to provide citizens with the living conditions necessary for health and well-being. As such, these policies also ensure societal well-being. The primary values shaping these approaches is, in the case of the social-democratic Scandinavian nations, the promotion of equality and, in the case of the continental European nations, the maintaining of solidarity.[4]

The role of values is also especially relevant when we consider the issue of poverty rates. In many nations, reducing poverty and promoting early child development is a central concern of governments and policy-makers at all levels. Based on collective action realized through public policy, these nations make a commitment to reducing the impacts of the risks (from adverse living conditions through unemployment, disability and illness, to retirement) that citizens experience across the lifespan. These approaches are far less common in Canada.

Public policy is therefore especially important for improving the quality of the socio-economic conditions and patterns that constitute the social determinants of health. Governments influence the distribution of income and other resources by setting — or not setting — employment standards, wage levels, and the nature and quality of benefits, and by determining whether these benefits are universal or targeted. Governments are responsible for housing and child-care policies, enacting retraining programs, and providing educational opportunities.

Some policies, such as providing an adequate income for all, would have an impact on a variety of the social determinants of health. Policies concerned with promoting a more equitable distribution of income would also respond to issues of housing and food insecurity, early child development, and social exclusion. Policies focused on increasing employment security and working conditions would likewise make a positive contribution to issues of income distribution, housing and food insecurity, early child development, and social exclusion (as we have seen in earlier chapters).

The common theme running through these proposed public policies is that they assist Canadians with managing risk and navigating the life-course. Health ethicist David Seedhouse says that to achieve health, in addition to adequate and responsive health care, people must be provided with: 1) resources to meet the basic needs of food, drink, shelter, warmth, and purpose in life; 2) access to the widest possible information about all factors that have an influence on a person's life; 3) skills of numeracy and literacy and the confidence to use this information; and 4) opportunities to be connected with others in their community and to the larger society.[5]

Mary Shaw and her colleagues at the University of Bristol specify that health-related public policy plays its greatest role in assisting people to navigate significant life-course transitions during which they are especially vulnerable to health disadvantage.[6] These moments include foetal development, nutritional growth and health in childhood, leaving home, entering the labour market, job loss or insecurity, and episodes of illness and treatment, among others. Material disadvantage and the absence of societal supports during these key periods work against health. The link between the navigation of these transitions and the impact of the varying social determinants of health is striking.

For example, foetal development, nutritional growth, and health in childhood are clearly linked to the availability of the social determinants of income, food, and housing; the transitions of entering the labour market, job loss, or insecurity are linked to employment security and working conditions; and episodes of illness are linked with the quality of the social safety net and health care.

The risks are of two types: universal risks, such as the life transitions identified by Shaw and colleagues; and non-universal risks, such as premature disease, injuries and accidents, and family breakups, among others. Societies individualize risk when they fail to provide public, collectively organized benefits and services to respond to these situations, or when they do not manage risk collectively through the universal provision of a basket of benefits and services. Collective approaches to managing risk are essential in meeting the needs of the majority of Canadians.

In particular, as Professor Gosta Esping-Andersen points out, managing risk during childhood is essential for a society to meet the demands of a post-industrial economy:

> There is one basic finding that overshadows all others, namely that remedial policies for adults are a poor (and

costly) substitute for interventions in childhood. Since a person's job and career prospects depend increasingly on his or her cognitive abilities, this is where it all begins. Activating or retraining adults is profitable and realistic if these same adults already come with a sufficient ability to learn. Households with limited resources can probably never be eradicated entirely, but their relative proportion can be minimized and this is our single greatest policy challenge.[7]

For Esping-Andersen, the primary factors shaping children's cognitive abilities are health, income poverty, and developmental priming mechanisms that set the stage for lifelong learning. Of foremost importance for achieving health and minimizing income poverty is, he maintains, the establishment of strong welfare states — and it is here that Canada appears to be sorely lagging — that provide security to their citizens. Esping-Andersen's analysis is consistent with the arguments that place their prime emphasis on the social determinants of health. When it comes to the developmental priming mechanisms, he sees the provision of universal high-quality child care in support of early child development as essential. As we have seen in earlier chapters, the evidence on how Canada is meeting these requirements is discouraging.

Population Health and Public Policy: The Indicators

Canada is among the wealthiest nations in the world. In terms of the size of the economy the average Canadian is annually worth U.S. $38,433, which places Canada seventh among thirty OECD nations. Given this relatively wealthy position, how do Canada's health indicators compare to other nations? Compared to the member nations of the OECD, on a number of population health indicators, Canada's ranks poorly.

Canada's ranking in life expectancy, though high, has been

Table 6-1. Selected Indicators of Canadian Health Outcomes in Comparison to the Wealthy Developed Nations of the Organisation for Economic Co-operation and Development

Health Indicator	Canada's Score	Canada's Ranking (1=best)
Life expectancy — total	80.2 years	9th of 30
Life expectancy — males	77.8 years	5th of 30
Life expectancy — females	82.6 years	9th of 30
Premature years of life lost prior to age 70 — males	4296/100,000	10th of 26
Premature years of life lost prior to age 70 — females	2669/100,000	18th of 27
Deaths from ischemic heart disease — males	134/100,000	13th of 27
Deaths from ischemic heart disease — females	62.7/100,000	14th of 27
Deaths from cancer	358/100,000	12th of 27
Deaths from cancer — males	213/100,000	12th of 27
Deaths from cancer — females	145/100,000	19th of 27
Infant mortality	5.3/1000	24th of 30
Low birth-weight rates	5.9/100	9th of 30
Child death by injury rates	97/100,000	18th of 26
Teenage live births	20.2/1000	21st of 28

Sources: Organisation for Economic Cooperation and Development, "Health at a Glance 2007," OECD Indicators Paris: Organisation for Economic Cooperation and Development, 2007; Innocenti Research Centre, "A League Table of Child Deaths by Injury in Rich Nations," and "A League Table of Teenage Births in Rich Nations," Florence: Innocenti Research Centre, 2001.

consistently slipping since the early 1990s. The recent history of the country's infant mortality rate, which is often identified as the most sensitive indicator of overall population health, is also telling. In 1980 Canada's infant mortality rate was 10 deaths per 1000 births, which gave it a relative ranking of tenth of thirty OECD nations. By 2005 Canada had improved that to 5.3/1000, a significant achievement, but that decline failed to match the pattern seen in other OECD nations — so much so that Canada's ranking over that period fell from tenth to twenty-fourth of thirty OECD nations.[8]

Most of the nations doing better than Canada in both infant mortality and low birth-weight rates are not as wealthy as Canada in terms of per capita gross domestic product (GDP). For example, the average Swede is worth U.S. $2,000 less than the average Canadian in terms of national per capita GDP, yet Sweden's health indicators such as life expectancy, infant mortality, and low birth-weight rate are far superior to those of Canada.

Canadian Public Policy in Comparative Perspective

Citizen Security

The level of citizen security is another important indicator of well-being, and total public expenditure is in turn a key indicator of a national commitment to the provision of citizen security. The best measure of this is the extent to which a nation collects revenues and transfers them to citizens in the form of various benefits, programs, and services. Such allocations include spending on education, employment training, social assistance, family supports, pensions, health and social services, and free or subsidized housing. In 2005 Canada allocated 16.5 percent of its GDP on such spending — which placed Canada twenty-fifth on a list of twenty-nine OECD nations. Nations such as Italy, Finland, Belgium, Germany, Denmark, Austria, France, and Sweden all allocate over 25 percent of their GDP on such public expenditures. The United States allocated 16 percent of its GDP towards these expenditures, just slightly behind Canada.

Income and Income Distribution

Interestingly, nations that spend less on public expenditures are also the ones with greater income and wealth inequalities — which has much to do with a governmental reluctance to implement policies that redistribute income and wealth, thus leaving it to the market to determine. The end result is growing inequality, and the inadequate provision of public services and supports has its inevitable reflection in the social determinants of health.

Income inequality in Canada has increased markedly since 1980, with the increase being especially great for market income. The OECD notes that Canada — together with Germany — showed the greatest increases in income inequality from the mid-1990s to the mid-2000s. In addition, Canada was above the average in income inequality. The reduction in inequality from the distributional effects of the tax and benefits system — which redistribute some income to lower-income people in Canada — fell well behind such effects seen in most other OECD nations.[9]

The percentage of Canadians living on low incomes from 1980

The Canadian Social Safety Net

"For years, we bragged that we were identified by the United Nations as 'the best country in the world in which to live.' We have since dropped a few ranks, but our bragging continues. We would be the most surprised to learn that, in all countries — and that includes Canada — health and illness follow a social gradient: the lower the socioeconomic position, the worse the health.

"The truth is that Canada — the ninth richest country in the world — is so wealthy that it manages to mask the reality of poverty, social exclusion and discrimination, the erosion of employment quality, its adverse mental health outcomes, and youth suicides. While one of the world's biggest spenders in health care, we have one of the worst records in providing an effective social safety net. What good does it do to treat people's illnesses, to then send them back to the conditions that made them sick?"

Source: The Hon. Monique Bégin, Former Minister of National Health and Welfare, fore-word to J. Mikkonen and D. Raphael, 2010, *Social Determinants of Health: The Canada Facts* <thecanadianfacts.org>.

to 2007 was on the rise.[10] That was the situation prior to the onset of the 2008 recession, and clearly, conditions have since deteriorated.

Moreover, among OECD nations Canada has one of the highest poverty rates for families with children. Indeed, Canada is one of the few nations in which child poverty rates were higher than overall poverty rates over the past two decades. Canada fares even worse in terms of the percentage of workers considered to be low-paid (defined as earning less than two-thirds of the median wage). As a Statistics Canada report notes, "Canada (24%) and the United States (23%) had the highest proportions of low-paid workers among the 12 countries for which data are available, with nearly 1 in 4 workers earning less than two-thirds of median annual earnings in 2000 and in 2004."[11] Compare this standing with Finland and Denmark, which have about 7 percent of employees identified in this category.

Education
In 2006 Canada spent 6.5 percent of GDP on education overall,[12] which placed it fifth among OECD nations. Canada did less well in terms of primary and secondary education, spending 3.7 percent of its GDP, giving it a rank of fourteenth of twenty-nine; whereas post-secondary spending, at 2.7 percent, placed Canada at second among twenty-eight OECD nations.

Unemployment and Employment Security
Canada's unemployment rate of 6.1 percent in 2008 was above the OECD average, giving it a rank of seventeenth of thirty OECD nations (in March of 2010 the corresponding figure was 8.3 percent). More importantly, the OECD calculates an employment protection index of rules and regulations that protect employment and provides benefits to temporary workers.[13] In that measurement Canada achieved a score that placed it at twenty-sixth of twenty-eight nations.

This abysmal picture of employment protection illustrates Canada's rather meagre allocations for what is termed "active labour policy" — public policy that strives to reduce unemployment through employment training and upgrading. Active labour policy is especially important in times of changing employment patters as a result of increasing economic globalization. Canada is ranked twenty-first among thirty OECD nations in such spending. In 1985 Canada spent almost .6 percent of GDP on such policies, but has since reduced that by half, to .3 percent.[14]

Employment and Working Conditions

Working conditions, benefits, and opportunities for advancement are strongly related to whether workers are covered by collective agreements and employed in unionized workplaces. In comparative perspective Canadian workers are less likely to have their wages and working conditions set by collective agreements.[15]

Collective agreements are not only commonplace among the Scandinavian nations, where union membership is high, but also among continental European nations, where union membership is lower. Much of this has to do with the business sector recognizing the need to work with governments and labour to ensure that citizens and workers are able to experience a decent quality of life. Although union membership is lower in those other European countries than it is in the Scandinavian nations, the unions there tend to be very militant. Such co-operation is rather less likely in nations identified as liberal political economies, such as the United Kingdom, United States, Canada, and New Zealand.

Early Childhood Development

Along with Canada's child poverty rate, which is amongst the highest of OECD nations, the country is also among the worst in meeting early childhood education and care benchmarks. Canadian families do not have access to regulated child-care spaces, which is not surprising given that Canada spends the lowest proportion of national resources on early child education and care among wealthy developed nations. Canada's spending exceeds only that of Greece.[16]

Figure 6-1. Public Expenditure on Child Care and Early Education Services, Percent of GDP, Selected OECD Nations, 2005

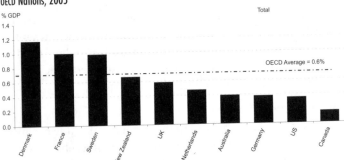

Source: Social Expenditure database 1980–2005; OECD Education database; US Department of Health and Human Services.

Food Security

The percentage of Canadians experiencing food insecurity is just over 9 percent. Comparative data on food security — or food poverty, as it is called in the United Kingdom — for other wealthy developed nations is only available for the English-speaking nations. In Australia and the United Kingdom, the rate of food insecurity is estimated at 5 percent. Not surprisingly, the figure for the United States is 12.6 percent. In New Zealand it is a striking 20 percent.[17]

Housing

In 2007, 21 percent of Canadians spent more than 30 percent of their income on housing costs, an excessive amount, according to CMHC.[18] Among renters the figure was a striking 35 percent, an increase from 31 percent in 1991. Canada is the only developed nation that does not have a national housing policy. Canada now spends .44 percent of its GDP on housing, which gives it a rank of eleventh of twenty-four OECD nations. The country faces a crisis of housing affordability.

Table 6-2. Selected International and Aboriginal HDI Scores, 2001

HDI Rank	Country	HDI Score
	Selected Countries with High Human Development	(0.800–1)
1	Norway	.944
2	Iceland	.942
3	Sweden	.941
7	United States	.937
8	**Canada**	**.937**
13	United Kingdom	.930
17	France	.925
20	New Zealand	.917
31	U.S. American Indian and Alaska Native	.877
33	**Canadian Aboriginal Population**	**.851**

Source: Adapted from M. Cooke et al., "Indigenous Well-Being in Four Countries: An Application of the UNDP's Human Development Index to Indigenous Peoples in Australia, Canada, New Zealand, and the United States," BMC International Health and Human Rights 7: 9, 2007.

Social Exclusion

As we've seen, according to the data, when it comes to their employment situations and wages, Aboriginal, racialized groups, women, and people with disabilities fare poorly as compared to those not in these groups.

Martin Cooke and his colleagues calculated Human Development Index (HDI) scores for indigenous peoples in Australia, Canada, New Zealand, and the United States and compared these to non-indigenous peoples in these nations and to other nations' overall scores.[19] HDI scores consist of an equal weighting of life expectancy, educational participation and adult literacy rates, with GDP per capita in constant dollars. While Canada ranked eighth overall in HDI scores, the index score for indigenous peoples ranked Canada at thirty-third.

Gender

In measurements of female wages as a percentage of male wages, Canada ranks nineteenth of twenty-one OECD countries, showing a gender wage gap of 21 percent (Figure 6-2).[20]

On another measurement of gender empowerment, which combines three domains — political participation and decision-making, economic participation and decision-making, and power over economic resources — in 2007 Canada ranked twelfth of twenty-four OECD nations.[21]

Figure 6-2. Gender Gap in Wages, Selected OECD Nations, in Percentage, 2006

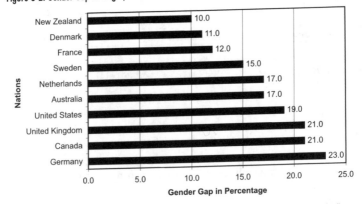

Source: Organisation for Economic Co-operation and Development (OECD), "Gender Gap in Median Earnings of Full-time Employees," <www.oecd.org/dataoecd/1/35/43199347.xls>, 2009.

Disability

Disability-related public policy can be divided into "benefits-related" policy and "integration-related" policy.[22] Benefits-related policy refers to the accessibility and generosity of benefits available to persons with disabilities, while integration-related policy refers to the extent to which persons with disabilities are provided with opportunities to participate in paid employment. Canada ranks amongst the lowest in benefit provision to people with disabilities and is well below the average in integration policy. Moreover, Canada is amongst the lowest spenders in what the OECD calls "incapacity spending," which refers to all the monies made available to provide benefits to persons with disabilities or to assist them in gaining employment.[23] Canada spends less than 1 percent of GDP, giving it a rank of eighteenth of twenty-three OECD nations.

Social Safety Net

Given all of these findings, it is not at all surprising that Canada also does very poorly when it comes to our much-vaunted social safety net. To take one example, Canada's unemployment benefits, which would be made available for someone experiencing unemployment for a five-year period, represent only 22 percent of the median wage — well below the OECD average, giving Canada a ranking of seventeenth of twenty-seven OECD nations.

Canada also performs poorly in terms of the social assistance benefits provided to those who are unable to work. Canada's social assistance for a lone parent with two children, for instance, is 37 percent of median household income, well below the poverty line.[24] For this family situation, Canada's benefits give it a ranking of twenty-second of twenty-nine OECD nations. A married couple with two children does not fare much better: Canada provides benefits equal to 32 percent of median household income, for an identical ranking of twenty-second of twenty-nine nations.

Health-Care Services

Canada's public spending on health care as a percentage of GDP is amongst the highest of OECD nations at 6.8 percent in 2006 for a rank of eighth of thirty OECD nations. Since public spending on health care is reflected in public health-care coverage, it is not surprising that all of the seven higher-spending nations cover a greater proportion of health-care costs than our system does. But of the thirty OECD nations, it is not just seven, but twenty-one nations that cover

Strengthening the Social Determinants of Health through Public Policy Action

Policies to reduce the incidence of low income
- Raise the minimum wage to a living wage.
- Improve pay equity.
- Restore and improve income supports for those unable to gain employment.
- Provide a guaranteed minimum income.

Policies to reduce social exclusion
- Enforce legislation that protects the rights of minority groups, particularly concerning employment rights and anti-discrimination.
- Ensure that families have sufficient income to provide their children with the means of attaining healthy development.
- Reduce inequalities in income and wealth within the population through progressive taxation of income and inherited wealth.
- Assure access to educational, training, and employment opportunities, especially for the long-term unemployed.
- Remove barriers to health and social services, which involves understanding where and why such barriers exist.
- Provide adequate follow-up support for those leaving institutional care.
- Create housing policies that provide enough affordable housing of reasonable standard.
- Institute employment policies that preserve and create jobs.
- Direct attention to the health needs of immigrants and to the unfavourable socio-economic position of many groups, including the particular difficulties that many new Canadians face in accessing health and other care services.

Policies to strengthen Canada's social infrastructure
- Restore health and service program spending to the average level of OECD nations.
- Develop a national housing strategy and allocate an additional 1 percent of federal spending for affordable housing.
- Provide a national day-care program.
- Provide a national pharmacare program.

- Restore eligibility for and the level of employment benefits to previous levels.
- Require that provincial social assistance programs be accessible and funded at levels to ensure health.
- Ensure that supports are available to support Canadians through critical life transitions.

Source: D. Raphael and A. Curry-Stevens, "Surmounting the Barriers: Making Action on the Social Determinants of Health a Public Policy Priority," in Raphael, D. (ed.), *Social Determinants of Health: Canadian Perspectives*, second edition, Toronto: Canadian Scholars' Press, 2009.

a greater proportion of total health-care costs than does Canada. Indeed, the percentage of health-care costs covered by Canada's medicare system is only 70 percent, which gives Canada a rank of twenty-second of thirty nations for public coverage of health-care costs. The health-care systems of the United Kingdom, Sweden, Czech Republic, Luxembourg, Denmark, Norway, Iceland, France, and Japan — all of which except France spend less public monies on health care than Canada does — cover more than 80 percent of health-care costs. The only nations in which coverage is lower than Canada are Slovakia, Australia, Netherlands, Greece, Switzerland, Korea, United States, and Mexico.

Governments, Markets, and Health

For many Canadians the social determinants of health have a grievous impact because of how the economic system acts to distribute resources so unequally. In addition, governments make matters worse by leaving what should be public policy — distribution of income and wealth, provision of benefits, supports, and services — to the market to determine. Compared to other wealthy developed nations, Canada falls far behind in managing its economic system in a way that provides citizens with a higher and more equitable quality of life, health, and well-being.

Short of a radical restructuring of our market-dominated socio-economic system, governments can do many things to deal with these deficiencies. The actions fall into three main areas: policies to reduce the incidence of lower-income, policies to reduce social exclusion, and policies to strengthen Canada's social infrastructure. These are all public policy goals that can be achieved. All we need is the political will to carry them out. In all likelihood, however, this project will only come about as a result of public mobilization in support of these efforts.

Notes

1. World Health Organization. 2008. *Closing the Gap in a Generation: Health Equity Through Action on the Social Determinants of Health.* Geneva: World Health Organization: p. 1.

2. Commission on Social Determinants of Health. 2005. "Towards a Framework for Analysis and Action on the Social Determinants of Health." Draft report, WHO Health Equity Team, Geneva. May <http://www.acphd.org/healthequity/healthequity/documents/WHOConceptualFrame-1.pdf>.

3. G. Esping-Andersen. 2009. *The Unfinished Revolution: Welfare State Adaptation to Women's New Roles.* Cambridge, UK: Polity Press.

4. S. Saint-Arnaud and P. Bernard. 2003. "Convergence or Resilience? A Hierarchical Cluster Analysis of the Welfare Regimes in Advanced Countries." *Current Sociology* 51 (5): 499–527.

5. D. Seedhouse. 2003. *Health: The Foundations of Achievement.* New York: John Wiley.

6. M. Shaw, D. Dorling, D. Gordon, and G.D. Smith. 1999. *The Widening Gap: Health Inequalities and Policy in Britain.* Bristol, UK: Policy Press.

7. G. Esping-Andersen. 2002. "A Child-Centred Social Investment Strategy." In G. Esping-Andersen (ed.), *Why We Need a New Welfare State.* Oxford UK: Oxford University Press: p. 19.

8. Robert Wood Johnson Foundation. 2008. *Overcoming Obstacles to Health.* Princeton: Robert Wood Johnson Foundation; Organisation for Economic Cooperation and Development. 2007. *Health at a Glance 2007.* OECD Indicators. Paris: OECD.

9. Statistics Canada. 2009. "Cansim Table 2020705. Gini Coefficients

of Market, Total and After-Tax Income, by Economic Family Type." Ottawa: Statistics Canada; Organisation For Economic Co-operation and Development (OECD). 2008. *Growing Unequal: Income Distribution and Poverty in OECD Nations.* Paris: OECD; Innocenti Research Centre. 2005. *Child Poverty in Rich Nations, 2005. Report Card No. 6.* Florence: Innocenti Research Centre; T. Smeeding. 2005. "Poor People in Rich Nations: The United States in Comparative Perspective." Syracuse, NY: Luxembourg Income Study Working Paper #419. Syracuse University, Syracuse.

10. Statistics Canada. 2009. "Cansim Table 2020802. Individuals in Low Income, by Economic Family Type, 2007 Constant Dollars." Ottawa: Statistics Canada.

11. International differences in low-paid work Sébastien LaRochelle-Côté and Claude Dionne June 2009 Perspectives 5 Statistics Canada — Catalogue no. 75-001-X

12. Organisation for Economic Co-operation and Development (OECD). 2009. "Education at a Glance 2009: OECD Indicators." <http://www.oecd.org/document/62/0,3343,en_2649_39263238_43586328_1_1_1_37455,00.html>.

13. Organisation for Economic Co-operation and Development (OECD). 2009. "Strictness of Employment Protection." <http://stats.oecd.org/Index.aspx?DataSetCode=EPL_OV>.

14. Organisation for Economic Co-operation and Development (OECD). 2009. "Social Expenditure Database." <http://stats.oecd.org/wbos/default.aspx?datasetcode=SOCX_AGG>.

15. Organization for Economic Cooperation and Development (OECD). 2006. "Trade Union Members and Union Density." <http://www.oecd.org/dataoecd/8/24/31781139.xls>; Organization for Economic Cooperation and Development (OECD). 2009. *Growing Unequal: Income Distribution and Poverty in OECD Countries.* Paris: OECD.

16. J. Beach et al. 2009. *Early Childhood Education and Care in Canada 2008.* Toronto: Childcare Resource and Research Unit; Organisation for Economic Co-operation and Development (OECD). 2009. <www.oecd.org/dataoecd/44/20/38954032.xls.>

17. J. Temple. 2008. "Severe and Moderate Forms of Food Insecurity: Are they Distinguishable?" *Australian Journal of Social Issues* 43: 649–68; M. Nord and H.A. Hopwood. 2008. *Comparison of Household Food Security in Canada and the United States.* Washington, DC: U.S. Dept. of Agriculture; C. McKerchar. 2006. "Food Security in New Zealand: A Very Brief

Overview." <www.ana.org.nz/documents/ChristinaMcKerchar.pdf>.

18. Canada Mortgage and Housing Corporation (CMHC). 2009. *Housing in Canada On-line.* <http://data.beyond2020.com/cmhc/HiCODefinitions_EN.html#_Affordable_dwellings_1>.

19. M. Cooke et al. 2007. "Indigenous Well-being in Four Countries: An Application of the UNDP's Human Development Index to Indigenous Peoples in Australia, Canada, New Zealand, and the United States." *BMC International Health and Human Rights* 7: 9.

20. Organisation for Economic Co-operation and Development (OECD). 2009. "Gender Gap in Median Earnings of Full-time Employees." <www.oecd.org/dataoecd/1/35/43199347.xls>.

21. Human Development Program. 2009. *Human Development Report.* <http://hdrstats.undp.org/en/indicators/126.html>.

22. Organisation for Economic Co-operation and Development (OECD). 2003. *Transforming Disability into Ability: Policies to Promote Work and Income Security for People with Disabilities.* Paris: OECD.

23. Organisation for Economic Co-operation and Development (OECD). 2009. "Social Expenditure Database." <http://stats.oecd.org/wbos/default.aspx?datasetcode=SOCX_AGG>.

24. Organisation for Economic Co-operation and Development (OECD). 2009. "Net Incomes of Social Assistance Recipients in Relation to Alternative Poverty Lines, 2007." <http://dx.doi.org/10.1787/706265650677>.

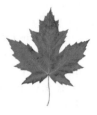

7. WHAT NEEDS TO BE DONE?

Improve the conditions of daily life — the circumstances in which people are born, grow, live, work, and age. Tackle the inequitable distribution of power, money, and resources — the structural drivers of those conditions of daily life — globally, nationally, and locally. —World Health Organization, *Closing the Gap*, 2008

Throughout the book, I have made various suggestions about the kinds of public policy that would make the distribution of resources in this country more equitable and have positive effects on the social determinants of health. These suggestions are not pipe dreams: they have been implemented to good effect in many wealthy industrialized nations, most of which are not as wealthy as Canada.

A commonly heard argument is that these nations accomplish health-promoting objectives at the expense of economic performance. However, the Conference Board of Canada's analysis of national performance based on indicators of health, health determinants, education and skills, environment, society, economy, and innovation found that the social-democratic nations not only outperformed Canada on most of the health and quality of life indicators, but also outperformed Canada on the economy and innovation indicators.[1]

But we do not only have to look to the nations that have adopted a social-determinants-of-health perspective. We can also look to the twenty-five years of Canada's history after the Great Depression and World War II, a period that saw the implementation of medicare and public pensions, the development of unemployment insurance, and federal and provincial programs that delivered affordable housing to Canadians. Like the overseas countries, Canada has also had the experience of developing public policies that promote health and well-being and prevent illness.

Since the mid-twentieth-century period Canada has moved away from providing citizens with the means of maintaining their health. Although policy-makers are well aware of the trends and possibilities for a different approach — Canadian government documents and reports have been analyzing and putting forth these ideas since the mid-1970s — Canada has come to be a laggard on the social determinants of health front. Much of this has to do with the concept being at odds with governmental approaches to public policy. If Canada is to return to a public policy pathway that focuses on the social determinants of health, we will need to build strong social and political movements that pressure governments and policy-makers to enact health-supporting measures and to avoid what the WHO calls "regressive societal phenomenon."

Moving Forward

Our different levels and institutions of governments would be more likely to focus policies and research on the role of the social determinants of health if they had evidence that public opinion was in favour of such action. But for the most part Canadians seem to be unaware that the primary determinants of health are their living conditions and social status and that governments have been failing to develop public policies that will alter the situation. A primary reason for this lack of public understanding is the preoccupation of governments, public health agencies, media, and disease associations with medical and individual lifestyle approaches to health and illness at the expense of a social determinants perspective. Any cursory review of institutional reports, public statements, and programs addressing health promotion and disease prevention will reveal these preoccupations. Meanwhile, an impressive number of scholars and researchers in universities across Canada have been studying the issues from a social perspective and attempting to communicate their findings and understandings to the general public.[2] Sadly, Canadians are not receiving the benefit of the extensive knowledge accumulated in hundreds of studies that detail the role of social conditions and factors as the primary contributors to health and primary cause of illness.

Still, increasing numbers of organizations and agencies in Canada have adopted a social determinants of health perspective. For these bodies, the evidence of the importance of the social determinants to their stakeholders and clients is so compelling that the issues cannot be ignored. These organizations and agencies should be encouraged to continue their efforts, and additional organizations should be engaged to follow their path. Unfortunately, their activities have had little influence upon public policy-making and certainly little penetration into Canadians' understanding of the causes of health and illness.

A social determinants of health agenda can thus be translated into health-supporting public policies through two main and interacting avenues. First, we need to educate and then mobilize Canadians to pressure governments and policy-makers to address the task of refocusing their efforts in a different direction — on the social determinants of health.

Second, we need to support candidates of political parties that are receptive to an approach based on the social determinants of health. These candidates can be found in every political party, but are more likely to be found and influenced in some political parties than in others. The candidates who are already open and genuinely interested in these ideas and issues should be supported, and those who are not particularly interested need to be pressured to adopt this new focus.

Canadians can act to implement a social determinants of health agenda as individuals or through their support of and/or membership in numerous advocacy groups. As individuals or supporters of these groups, people can make efforts to influence governments and policy-makers directly through lobbying activities or indirectly through ongoing public education that emphasizes and details the importance of the social determinants of health.

We should also direct efforts towards pressuring target institutions that have influence with governments and policy-makers. These institutions include local and provincial public health units, disease associations and their affiliates, and the media. Given their mandates of promoting the public's health, preventing disease, and informing their readership, there is every good reason that these institutions should be part of a social determinants of health movement.

Educating Canadians

Canadians are woefully uninformed about the social determinants of health.[3] When asked by surveys to provide the various means of maintaining health, Canadians overwhelmingly repeat the healthy-living mantra of diets, physical activity, rest, and avoidance of tobacco as the keys to good health. In no case has a majority of Canadians in a survey reported *any* social determinant of health as a significant influence upon health. This should not be surprising considering the ongoing barrage of health-lifestyle messages that Canadians are subjected to. The media's profound neglect of the social determinants of health contributes to this lack of knowledge.

How can Canadians be educated about the social determinants of health and then be encouraged to shape public policy? Perhaps the first step of an educational process is simply to pass the word: to tell friends, relatives, neighbours, and colleagues about the existence of social determinants and what this means for health. The resources that are available to assist in this task all communicate the same message: the primary determinants of health are not the "healthy lifestyle choices" that Canadians make, but rather the living conditions to which they are exposed, and the quality of these conditions are shaped by public policy decisions.

Alongside the word-of-mouth approach, we should insist that established communication systems that now convey "healthy lifestyle choices" instead bring their messages to the service of the social determinants of health. Public health units, disease associations, and government ministries of health expend tens of millions of dollars annually on such systems.[4] They must be urged to modify their

---

Canadian Understandings of the Determinants of Health

A sample representing the total population of Canadians was asked the following open-ended question: If you had to identify the three most important factors that contribute to GOOD health, what would they be? The responses were:

Diet/Nutrition:	82%
Physical Activity	70%
Proper Rest	13%
Not Smoking	12%

When provided with a list of various factors, the percentages of Canadians identifying the social determinants as having a strong or very strong impact were:

Whether a person has a job	49%
Child's early experiences	44%
A person's level of income	33%
A person's level of education	33%
Availability of quality housing	34%

Source: Canadian Population Health Initiative, *Select Highlights on Public Views of the Determinants of Health*, Ottawa, CPHI, 2004.

communications. Instead of speaking only of their previously used threats to health of "tobacco use," "unhealthy diets," and "lack of physical activity," they should be persuaded to include or substitute terms such as "unhealthy living conditions," "insecure living conditions," "unhealthy workplaces," or "difficult childhoods."

Shifting Health Messages to a Social Determinants of Health Perspective

Contrast these two sets of messages from the United Kingdom. The first set is typical of public health messages in Canada and elsewhere. The second offers an ironic version based on a social determinants of health perspective.

The traditional ten tips for better health
1. Don't smoke. If you can, stop. If you can't, cut down.
2. Follow a balanced diet with plenty of fruit and vegetables.
3. Keep physically active.
4. Manage stress by, for example, talking things through and making time to relax.
5. If you drink alcohol, do so in moderation.
6. Cover up in the sun, and protect children from sunburn.
7. Practice safer sex.
8. Take up cancer screening opportunities.
9. Be safe on the roads: follow the Highway Code.
10. Learn the First Aid ABCs: airways, breathing, circulation. (Liam Donaldson, 1999)

The social determinants ten tips for better health
1. Don't be poor. If you can, stop. If you can't, try not to be poor for long.
2. Don't have poor parents.
3. Be able to own a car.
4. Don't work in a stressful, low-paid manual job.
5. Don't live in damp, low-quality housing.
6. Be able to afford to go on a foreign holiday and sunbathe.
7. Practice not losing your job and don't become unemployed.

8. Take up all benefits you are entitled to, if you are unemployed, retired or sick or disabled.

9. Don't live next to a busy major road or near a polluting factory.

10. Learn how to fill in the complex housing benefit/asylum application forms before you become homeless and destitute. (David Gordon, 1999)

Source: L. Donaldson, "Ten Tips for Better Health," and D. Gordon, "An Alternative Ten Tips for Better Health," reprinted in D. Raphael (ed.), *Social Determinants of Health: Canadian Perspectives*, Second edition, Toronto: Canadian Scholars' Press, 2009.

Public Health Units

Public health units — with some notable exceptions — have been remarkably reluctant to communicate information about the social determinants of health to Canadians.

This deep-rooted ambivalence towards the social determinants of health is particularly apparent in the number of public health conferences and public health association documents whose titles suggest an immersion in concepts related to the social determinants of health — titles that contrast sharply with the actual activities carried out by public health authorities across Canada.

In actual practice, most public health units make little effort to communicate information about the social determinants of health to Canadians, and most do not consider it their role to advise governmental authorities and policy-makers when their proposed public policies threaten the quality of social conditions or skew the distribution of valuable resources. An example of this phenomenon occurred over ten years ago when a medical officer of health working in a large Canadian jurisdiction stated that raising issues of public policy and their contribution to health would result in a reduction of the agency's funding. Similar sentiments were expressed at a more recent meeting of health officials in Ontario. As a consultant to numerous public health and health-care agencies and institutions, I have repeatedly been told that raising public policy issues can be a "career-threatening move." Even faculty at university health sciences departments frequently tell me of their reluctance to raise these kinds of issues until after they receive academic tenure.

Public health units need to be assured that looking after the public's health will not lead to adverse consequences for them, Numerous public health units have been able to carry out these activities without incurring repercussions, yet the public health establishment and most local health units continue to struggle with how to deal with the social determinants of health. Unfortunately, the result of this struggle has been a general failure on the part of the public health community to inform Canadians about the social determinants of health; and a failure to influence governmental policy-makers to address the pertinent issues.

The exceptions certainly merit our recognition and support. A number of health units have taken on the task of applying the social determinants of health approach towards citizen education and have made related efforts to influence governmental policy-making. If you see the name of your local health unit listed among the names of these public health units (see Appendix), find out more about their activities and make sure to contact the staff or Board of Health members — both elected representatives and citizen members — to tell them that their efforts and activities are appreciated.

If your local health unit is not among those listed, inquire about the efforts it has undertaken to: a) inform community members about the social determinants of health; and b) influence governments and policy-makers to implement public policies based on the social determinants approach. If health unit staff and board members appear to be unaware of these concepts, direct them to the available resources. If they are aware of these concepts but have failed to act upon them, direct their attention to public health units that have applied these concepts in public health practice and demand similar efforts.

The most important things you need to know about *your health* may not be as obvious as you think.

Health = A rewarding job with a living wage
Little control at work, high stress, low pay, or unemployment all contribute to poor health.
Your job makes a difference.

Health = Food on the table and a place to call home
Having access to healthy, safe, and affordable food and housing is essential to being healthy.
Access to food and shelter makes a difference.

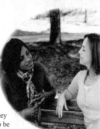

Health = Having options and opportunities
The thing that contributes most to your health is how much money you have. More money means having more opportunities to be healthy.
Money makes a difference.

Health = A good start in life
Prenatal and childhood experiences set the stage for lifelong health and well-being.
Your childhood makes a difference.

Health = Community belonging
A community that offers support, respect, and opportunities to participate helps us all be healthy.
Feeling included makes a difference.

How can you make a difference?
Action to improve the things that make
ALL of us healthy depends on ALL of our support.

Start a conversation.
Share what you know.

**To learn more, call the
Sudbury & District Health Unit
at (705) 522-9200, ext. 515
or visit www.sdhu.com.**

Make it a
Healthy
Day!
Sudbury & District Health Unit
Service de santé publique de Sudbury et du district

Disease Associations

If we just followed the advice of the major disease associations such as the Heart and Stroke Association, Canadian Diabetes Association, and Canadian Cancer Society, we would have no sense at all that social conditions and factors play a role in the incidence of the major life-ending diseases. Additionally, Canadians are assured that the major causes of cardiovascular disease, diabetes, and a host of other afflictions can be averted through the adoption of "healthy lifestyle choices." Even more importantly, Canadians are told that the solutions to these problems will come from medical and behavioural research rather than from public policy that improves the quality of and the distribution of the social determinants of health.

Not only do the messages of traditional disease associations ignore the direct role of the social determinants of health, but they also ignore how the social determinants themselves determine whether such "healthy lifestyle choices" are even possible for those most vulnerable to these diseases. Perhaps even more telling is the lack of consistent research evidence that these "healthy lifestyle choices" are reliable predictors of the onset of the chronic diseases, about which Canadians are understandably confused: not eating fruits and vegetables is sometimes found to be related to cardiovascular disease but not cancer, sometimes to cancer, but not cardiovascular disease, sometimes both, sometimes neither.

Disease association authorities need to be reminded that a primary cause of most of these chronic diseases can be traced to the social determinants of health. Even in cases in which the social determinants of health are not the primary cause of disease, such as with genetically determined diseases — Huntington's chorea or muscular dystrophy are two examples — it is still the prevailing social determinants of health that profoundly shape the lives of those so afflicted.

When experiencing the presence of a life-threatening or disabling disease — regardless of the causes — Canadian individuals

Major Disease Associations that Should Be Encouraged to Adopt a Social Determinants of Health Perspective

Alzheimer Society Canada*
Amyotrophic Lateral Sclerosis Society of Canada
The Arthritis Society*
The Brain Injury Association of Canada*
Canadian Breast Cancer Foundation
Canadian Cancer Society*
Canadian Cystic Fibrosis Foundation
Canadian Diabetes Association*
Canadian Foundation for AIDS Research*
Canadian Hospice Palliative Care Association
Canadian Liver Foundation*
Canadian Lung Association*
Canadian Mental health Association*
Canadian Orthopaedic Foundation
Crohn's and Colitis Foundation of Canada
Easter Seals Canada
The Foundation Fighting Blindness — Canada
Heart and Stroke Foundation of Canada*
Huntington Society of Canada
Kidney Cancer Canada
Lupus Canada*
The Kidney Foundation of Canada*
The Mood Disorders Society of Canada*
Muscular Dystrophy Canada
Multiple Sclerosis Society of Canada
Osteoporosis Canada*
Ovarian Cancer Canada
Parkinson Society Canada
SMARTRISK*
Spina Bifida and Hydrocephalus Association of Canada

* Identifies illnesses whose incidence is strongly associated with social determinants of health.

and families are increasingly faced with health and social services of deteriorating quality, a lack of financial supports, and increasing difficulty achieving secure and well-paying employment, among other problems. At the very minimum, disease associations should recognize that deteriorating social conditions cause great harm to families facing the presence of the illnesses around which these organizations are organized.

The implications of this analysis are obvious: disease associations that have influence with governments, policy-makers, and the public — and frequently have rather extensive resources — can join in advancing the social determinants of health agenda.

Why have these organizations not taken action? The most benign explanation may be that like Canadians in general they have been so subjected to lifestyle messages that they honestly do not know about the social determinants of health. Another may be that while they know about the social determinants of health as the primary causes of many of the diseases they are pledging to eliminate, they worry that raising the issues will alienate their corporate sponsors and public donors.

Why go out on a limb to raise issues that may threaten the agency when governments seem so unlikely to act upon these issues anyway? Finally, many members of the disease association's boards of directors come from the corporate and medical world and are not receptive to a social determinants of health message.

Nevertheless, if there is any hope of seriously promoting the health of Canadians, these disease associations, like public health units across Canada, must become strong advocates of the social determinants of health approach.

The Media

The media's coverage of health issues is narrow. Most often the focus is upon health care (for example, wait times, viral pandemics), biomedical research (isolation of disease genes, disease treatments) and health-related behaviours (diet, physical activity, and tobacco and alcohol use). Canada is not alone in this trend: Australia, the Netherlands, and the United Kingdom also show evidence of a narrow media coverage of health issues.[5] An extensive analysis of media stories in major Canadian newspapers over an eight-year period showed disheartening results.[6] The analysis of 4,732 newspaper articles concerned with health topics found a virtual blackout of stories concerned with the social determinants of health. Only 282 newspaper stories — 6 percent — were concerned with the socioeconomic environment. More specifically, only nine stories (well below one percent) were concerned with how income — the *primary* social determinant of health — is related to health. There is no reason to think that radio and television coverage is any different.

In a follow-up study, another team of researchers interviewed twelve Canadian newspaper health reporters about how they went about reporting health stories.[7] Not surprisingly, they found that most health reporters had a rudimentary understanding of the social determinants of health and were far from convinced that the social determinants of health represented a topic worth reporting. The reasons given by the reporters included: a) lack of knowledge of the social determinants on their part; b) difficulty putting the social determinants into the immediate and concrete "storytelling" that makes up typical news reporting; c) a perception that the social determinants were not new and therefore not newsworthy; and d) concern about "stigmatizing the poor."

I would add that most media outlets — including newspapers — are now owned by large corporate entities whose ideologies and values are not consistent with a social determinants of health perspective. Most reporters are probably well aware of this, and like most other salaried workers they hesitate to put their futures on the line by consistently presenting a social determinants of health perspective in their stories.

Clearly, there needs to be a systematic effort to shift how the Canadian media cover health issues. Citizens have an important role to play by writing letters to editors, health reporters, and columnists about the narrow health reporting and why the media need to communicate the ever-expanding social determinants of health research literature to their readers. But the public cannot accomplish this alone. Public health agencies, disease associations, professional health associations such as the Canadian Medical Association,[8] Canadian Nurses Association, and Canadian Public Health Association, and others concerned with promoting health must bring a concerted pressure to bear upon the media in order to bring about a sea change in reporting. Since most of these organizations have not consistently done so to date — the CNA being one exception — they will have to be encouraged to do so by their members and by us, their constituents and clients.

Another means of communicating the social determinants of health message may be through alternative media. The Social Determinants of Health Listserv, for example, run out of York University, provides a forum for over 1,200 members concerned with these issues.[9] Organizations such as moveon.org in the United States have been successful in having numerous issues taken up by governments and policy-makers. Is there space in Canada for the alternative media to set out a social determinants of health agenda? Certainly, stimulating the establishment of alternative media activities would be another step along the right path.

Mobilizing Canadians

Once educated about its importance, Canadians require a means of having this knowledge applied in the service of developing and implementing public policies that would address the social determinants of health and their related health outcomes. Clearly, to date, Canadian governments have been under little if any pressure to take this action. How can this be made to happen?

The answer to this question requires reflection about the means available for Canadians to have their concerns and interests met by agencies, institutions, governments, and policy-makers. In a democratic society, responsiveness to citizen concerns is to be expected. But as the objective quality of the social patterns and structures that shape health has deteriorated, and the distribution of resources has become more inequitable in Canada, it appears that many societal institutions have become less rather than more responsive to citizen concerns.

Political economists have argued that modern developed nations have characteristic ways of addressing public policy issues that are rooted in how their economic and political systems are organized. Why is it that the Scandinavian nations have public health and public policy approaches that focus on the social determinants of health while Canada, the United States, and, until recently, the United Kingdom do rather less in this regard? The answer may lie in what has been termed the "worlds of welfare" analysis of the roots of public policy.

Worlds of Welfare and the Social Determinants of Health

Gosta Esping-Andersen has identified various forms that the welfare state takes in advanced wealthy nations.[10] His "worlds of welfare" analysis indicates that Canada, the United States, United Kingdom, and Ireland constitute a cluster of nations identified as "liberal welfare states." Liberal welfare states provide the least support and security to their citizens and show the worst health profiles in terms of life expectancy and infant mortality rates. Canada's public policy profile is consistently found to be closer to that of the United States than to European welfare states, where citizen security and support are more ensured.

In contrast, nations such as Denmark, Norway, Finland, and Sweden are identified as "social-democratic welfare states." These nations provide the most support and security to their citizens and, not surprisingly, show the best health profiles. Nations identified as "conservative welfare states (Belgium, France, Germany, Netherlands) and "Latin welfare states" (Greece, Italy, Portugal) generally provide greater economic and social security to their citizens than do liberal welfare states.

In comparative terms, liberal welfare states, which provide the least support and security to their citizens, are dominated by an ideology of *liberty*, which calls for minimal government intervention in the workings of the marketplace. Indeed, such interventions are seen as providing a disincentive to work, thereby breeding "welfare dependence." The results of this ideological inspiration are meagre benefits provided to those on social assistance, generally weaker legislative support for the labour movement, underdeveloped policies for assisting those with disabilities, and reluctance to provide universal services and programs. Programs that exist are residual, which means that they exist to meet the most basic needs of the most deprived.

This approach primarily represents the interests of the corporate sector, the wealthy, and the well-established medical-industrial complex. It is no accident that these liberal welfare states have the greatest degree of wealth and income inequality, the weakest safety nets, and poorest performance based on indicators of population health such as infant mortality and life expectancy.

The social-democratic welfare states are just the opposite. The ideological inspiration for the central institution of these nations — the state — is *equity* realized through the reduction of poverty, inequality, and unemployment. Rather than seeing government responsibility as being limited to meeting the most basic needs of the most deprived, these nations take up as an organizing principle the concept of universalism, the provision of social rights for all citizens. Denmark, Finland, Norway, and Sweden are the best exemplars of this form of the welfare state. Governments with social-democratic political economies are proactive in identifying social problems and issues. They strive to promote citizens' economic and social security.

Compared to the liberal welfare states, the conservative and Latin welfare states generally provide superior economic and social security to their citizens, but they do so in terms of supporting families through the provision of supports for the principal wage-earner. The ideological inspiration of *solidarity* is achieved by promoting social stability, wage stability, and social integration.

Given these distinctions and their importance in public policy, it becomes clear that we need a change in political culture in Canada. Achieving that goal is the primary work of advocacy groups. Another means of doing so is by electing representatives who will be responsive to the implementation of a social determinants approach.

Advocacy Groups

Canada has numerous groups whose purpose is to influence governments and policy-makers to institute specific public policies. In these efforts, the groups also work to influence public opinion (that is, to educate Canadians and to change our political culture). Many of these groups focus directly or indirectly on the social determinants of health. The organizations try to connect Canadians with the latest information about these issues through newsletters and documents and reports. Canadians with knowledge of the social determinants of health and commitment to organizing around that perspective — to make the distribution more equitable — can join and/or support these groups.

Some organizations take the approach of supporting progressive public policy in general. These organizations in essence deal with a wide range of social determinants. Others are focused on specific social determinants of health (see Appendix).

Organizations such as the Canadian Centre for Policy Alternatives (CCPA) are concerned with a wide range of public policy issues that have strong affinities with the social determinants of health approach. It publishes the monthly *CCPA Monitor* as well as numerous research reports on issues such as pensions, income inequality and poverty, housing, and health care, among others. Anti-poverty groups such as Campaign 2000 and Canada without Poverty also deal with public policy issues such as income and its distribution, food security, housing, and child care.

Many organizations concern themselves with a specific social determinant of health such as food security, housing, or health care. Others focus on a specific health-related issue such as poverty among Canadians of colour, women with disabilities, women's health, or delivering health care to especially vulnerable Canadians. All of these organizations deserve the support of Canadians who are concerned about how the social determinants relate to the population's health and well-being. They can be a useful means of getting governments and policy-makers to respond to these issues.

The Media

It is unclear as to whether the major news sources can be brought around to a position where they will routinely write about the social determinants of health. Nevertheless, health reporters must be pressured to balance their health coverage, and when such reporting does occur, the rest of us should undertake immediate reinforcement in the form of letters to the editor and communications to the specific reporter. This kind of pressure has to be relentless, given the political economy of the mainstream media.

In my experience, columnists and social policy reporters are receptive to stories about the social determinants of health. It may also be that smaller, more local newspapers are a better avenue to have these issues raised. The alternative media may be more responsive, but also have smaller audiences. Whether the alternative media can fill the void left by the mainstream media is uncertain. Certainly, efforts directed towards target organizations such as public health and disease-oriented associations should include a request that they fully engage the media in the new messages they are putting forth about the social determinants of health.

Electoral Tactics

Every Canadian has an elected representative at the municipal, provincial/territorial, and federal level. These individuals are responsible for developing public policy that is responsive to Canadians' needs. Almost every day these various levels of government address issues related to health and the social determinants. Even when a government does not have a particular issue of that type, it can lobby other government levels to enact policies or programs. For examples, cities can lobby provincial governments to enact legislation that improves employment security and working conditions.

Identify your elected representative at each level and examine his or her personal position — as well as the party's position — on issues related to the social determinants of health. It may very well be that these people will not see the questions raised as health issues. If that is the case, direct their attention to the available material about the social determinants of health and indicate that your future support will depend on the policy position taken.

Political Parties

There are numerous reasons as to why anyone truly concerned about the social determinants of health should engage with Canada's political parties. The first is that every political party puts forth policy positions that revolve around those pertinent questions.

While there is ongoing concern about the failure of political parties to follow through on many of their campaign positions once they achieve power, a party's statement of positions does at least provide insight about what *might* be expected in the form of public policy if the party gains power. And if the party does not follow through, it can be held to account in the next election.

The second reason for engaging with political parties is that clear evidence is emerging that wealthy industrialized nations ruled by social-democratic parties of the left — and also to some extent conservative parties that are truly progressive and not of the current North American variety — are more likely to produce public policy that strengthens the quality of the social determinants of health.[11] This has especially been shown to be the case in the Scandinavian countries.

Professional Organizations, Employee Associations, and Unions

Many Canadians belong to employment-related associations, such as unions and professional associations, business associations such as chambers of commerce, and even employer associations such as school boards, children's aid societies, and others. Not only do many of these associations have nothing to say about the social determinants of health, but some even work against a social determinants agenda.

These associations have the means and the ability to issue statements and calls for governments to address issues related to the social determinants of health. Some of these associations have specific affinities to the perspective if their members are physicians, nurses, psychologists, educators, public health workers, social workers, municipal service employees, immigration workers, and early childhood education and care workers, among others. But all employment associations should be concerned with the social determinants of health as they affect the health and quality of life of all Canadians. With sufficient pressure from members, these associations could help advance a social determinants of health agenda.

Changing How Canada Is Run

The grievously harmful social determinants of health result in large part from the manner in which Canada's economic system — with the political system's endorsement — distributes resources amongst Canadians. In recent years Canada's institutions have become increasingly unresponsive to the needs of Canadians. Incomes of most Canadians are stagnating, and employment is becoming increasingly insecure. Social assistance and disability benefits lag behind inflation rates, pushing the most disadvantaged into even deeper conditions of deprivation. Food and housing insecurity is increasing. Social exclusion among vulnerable groups grows.

The economic system operates in such a manner that significant numbers of people are denied access to the living conditions that are necessary for proper health and well-being. Governments fail to intervene to address this state of affairs. The people responsible for this situation must be called to account. The counterbalances — labour unions, citizen groups, civil society organizations, and others — must be strengthened.

We have to engage and oppose those whose ideologies and values would turn Canada from *a society with a market-based economy* to *a market-driven society*.[12] We only need look to our neighbour to the

Making a Difference

Karen White's just like you. She works in client care for Bell Aliant, which she has done for over six years. But unlike the Bell Mobility Call Centre in Mississauga, Karen's workplace is unionized.

'There are so many benefits of having a union, I don't know where to start,' says the 31-year-old from Newfoundland. 'We get pay progressions every six months until we reach the top of our wage scale, as well as negotiated annual increases. They are all the same, everyone gets them and the manager doesn't get to play favourites.'

The pay is just the tip of the iceberg. 'If I'm sick, I still get paid, day, evening and weekend shift work has to be shared evenly amongst all employees, a regular (or permanent) worker can't be laid off if our work is outsourced, and schedules have to be posted four weeks in advance,' she explains. 'The last one offers real "work–life balance," to borrow one of Bell's terms.'

When it comes to career advancement, White says she has access to all the positions that come open.

'If I wanted to apply for an open job, I know that the company has to decide who to hire based on qualifications and seniority,' she explains. 'There are rules, the process is transparent and fair, and the managers are held accountable for the hiring decisions they make.'

Source: MobilityUnion, "'A Union Can Make a Difference in Your Life,' Says Nfld Bell Aliant Worker," 2010, <http://tinyurl.com/yetefwk>.

south to see what the cost of this transformation will be in terms of social inequality, disease and illness, and social disintegration.

Canadians must understand that the determinants of health and illness are primarily political, economic, and social issues — not medical conditions or lifestyle choices. The incidence and distribution of disease and illness are intimately tied up with how a society is organized and run. Health inequalities result from social inequalities. As Canadians come to understand this, the likelihood of governments and policy-makers enacting public policies that will promote health and prevent disease will increase. It is my hope that this book will serve as a call to action that will help to shift us towards that crucial goal.

Notes

1. Conference Board of Canada. 2003. *Defining the Canadian Advantage.* Ottawa: Conference Board of Canada; Conference Board of Canada. 2006. *Performance and Potential: The World and Canada.* Ottawa: Conference Board of Canada. The indicators include GDP per capita, GDP growth, productivity growth, unit labour cost, growth, inflation, deficit to GDP ratio, employment growth, unemployment rate, and long-term unemployment rate. Innovation indicators include spending on research and development, technological cooperation, patents in a range of areas, among others.

2. See the articles in the collection *Practising Public Scholarship: Experiences and Possibilities Beyond the Academy* for an exploration of the responsibility of academic scholars to their communities. <http://ca.wiley.com/WileyCDA/WileyTitle/productCd-1405189126.html>.

3. Canadian Population Health Initiative (CPHI). 2004. *Select Highlights on Public Views of the Determinants of Health.* Ottawa: CPHI.

4. See *The 2007 Report on the Integrated Pan-Canadian Healthy Living Strategy* to get a sense of the enormous amount of resources expended in "healthy living" activities in Canada. <http://www.phac-aspc.gc.ca/hl-vs-strat/pancan/pdf/pancan07-eng.pdf>. The Ontario Ministry of Health Promotion — heavily focused on diet, activity, and tobacco use — itself spends $7 million annually <http://www.fin.gov.on.ca/en/budget/estimates/2009-10/volume1/MHP.pdf>.

5. M. Bartley. 1995. "Medicine and the Media: Deprived of health." *BMJ* 310 (6978): 539; M.J. Commers, G. Visser, and E. De Leeuw. 2000. "Representations of Preconditions for and Determinants of Health in the Dutch Press." *Health Promotion International* 15 (4): 321–32; B. Westwood, and G. Westwood. 1998. "Assessment of Newspaper Reporting of Public Health and the Medical Model: A Methodological Case Study." *Health Promotion International* 14 (1): 53–64.

6. M. Hayes et al. 2007. "Telling Stories: News Media, Health Literacy and Public Policy in Canada." *Social Science and Medicine* 54: 445–57.

7. M. Gasher et al. 2007. "Spreading the News: Social Determinants of Health Reportage in Canadian Daily Newspapers." *Canadian Journal of Communication* 32 (3): 557–74.

8. While it might be suggested that a medical association such as the CMA would have a vested interest in promulgating a medical perspective on health issues, we should take them at their word that they are committed to promoting health and preventing disease. See <http://policybase. cma.ca/PolicyPDF/PD04-06.pdf>.

9. To join the list, send the following message to listserv@yorku.ca: subscribe sdoh *yourfirstname yoursecondname.*

10. G. Esping-Andersen. 1990. *The Three Worlds of Welfare Capitalism.* Princeton: Princeton University Press.

11. A. Alesina and E.L. Glaeser. 2004. *Fighting Poverty in the US and Europe: A World of Difference.* Toronto: Oxford University Press; L. Rainwater and T.M. Smeeding. 2003. *Poor Kids in a Rich Country: America's Children in Comparative Perspective.* New York: Russell Sage Foundation; D. Brady. 2003. "The Politics of Poverty: Left Political Institutions, the Welfare State, and Poverty." *Social Forces* 82: 557–88.

12. E. Broadbent. 2009. "Barbarism Lite: The Political Attack on Social Rights." *Toronto Star* February 21. <www.thestar.com/comment/article/590845>.

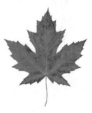

APPENDIX

Key Resources on the Social Determinants of Health in Canada

Policy and Advocacy Organizations Addressing the Social Determinants of Health

The Canadian Centre for Policy Alternatives — www.policyalternatives.ca

The Caledon Institute of Social Policy — www.caledoninst.org

The Wellesley Institute — http://wellesleyinstitute.com

National Aboriginal Health Organization — www.naho.ca

Campaign 2000 — www.campaign2000.ca

Canada without Poverty www.cwp-csp.ca/Blog

The Childcare Resource and Research Unit — www.childcarecanada.org

The Child Care Advocacy Association of Canada — www.ccaac.ca/home.php

The Disabled Women's Network — http://dawn.thot.net

The ODSP Action Coalition — www.odspaction.ca

Ethno-Racial People with Disabilities Coalition of Ontario — www.ryerson.ca/erdco

The Canadian Labour Congress — www.canadianlabour.ca

The Institute for Work & Health — www.iwh.on.ca

Food Secure Canada — http://foodsecurecanada.org

Food Banks Canada — http://foodbankscanada.ca

The Toronto Disaster Relief Committee — www.tdrc.net

The Cooperative Housing Federation — www.fhcc.coop/eng/pages2007/home.asp
The Colour of Poverty — www.colourofpoverty.ca.
The Canadian Women's Health Network — www.cwhn.ca
The Ontario Women's Health Network — www.owhn.on.ca

Health Units

British Columbia: Vancouver Coastal Health; Interior Health Authority
Alberta: Chinook
Saskatchewan: Regina; Saskatoon
Ontario: Hamilton; London; North Bay; Parry Sound District; Ottawa; Perth; Peterborough; Sudbury; Waterloo
Quebec: Montreal
Nova Scotia: Guysborough Antigonish-Strait Health Authority
Newfoundland and Labrador: Western Region

Media Resources

"Poor no More" (2010) — www.poornomore.ca
"Population Health: The New Agenda" (2009) Vancouver Coastal Health Unit. — www.lemongrassmedia.net/lgm/blog/files/pophealth-the-new-agenda.html
"Sick People or Sick Societies?" (2008). *CBC Ideas.* — http://tinyurl.com/yg5tk38 and http://tinyurl.com/yksyl56
"Unnatural Causes: Is Inequality Making us Sick?" (2008). *California Newsreel.* — Available at www.unnaturalcauses.org.

Website Resources

Canadian Public Health Association Policy Statements — www.cpha.ca/en/programs/policy.aspx
Dennis Raphael's Website — www.atkinson.yorku.ca/draphael
Public Health Agency of Canada — www.phac-aspc.gc.ca/ph-sp/approach-approche/index-eng.php
Social Determinants of Health: The Canadian Facts — www.thecanadianfacts.org
WHO Commission on Social Determinants of Health — www.who.int/social_determinants/en/

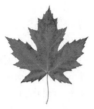

ACKNOWLEDGEMENTS

One of the greatest pleasures of my professional life has been the opportunity to meet and work with committed researchers and policy advocates from across Canada — people from the wide range of sectors that have come to be known as representing the social determinants of health. Much of this book represents an integration and synthesis of their work, and I have made every attempt to recognize and communicate their contributions.

These individuals include Carolyne Alix, Pat Armstrong, Nathalie Auger, Toba Bryant, Tracey Burns, Fernando Cartwright, Ann Curry-Stevens, Janice Foley, Martha Friendly, Grace-Edward Galabuzi, Lars Hallstrom, Andrew Jackson, Ronald Labonte, David Langille, Elizabeth McGibbon, Lynn McIntyre, Michael Polanyi, Krista Rondeau, Barbara Ronson, Irving Rootman, Michael Shapcott, Peter Smith, Brenda L. Smith-Chant, Janet Smylie, Emile Tompa, Diane-Gabrielle Tremblay, Valerie Tarasuk, and Charles Ungerleider.

All of these people practise what University of Washington professor Katharyne Mitchell calls public scholarship. They recognize the need to move their research findings and recommendations beyond the academy in the service of influencing the making of public policy. Their activities have promoted better understandings of what needs to be done. Indeed, a simple Google search of any of these individuals will document the extent of their efforts.

But to date our attempts to prod our governments and elected representatives to implement health-promoting public policy have fallen well short of what is being accomplished in other nations. This book is one more attempt to move this agenda forward and I am very appreciative of Fernwood Publishing — especially Wayne Anthony and Beverley Rach — and the others involved in this project — Robert Clarke, Debbie Mathers, and Brenda Conroy — for their support of this effort. In these dark times, it will do us well to recall that Tommy Douglas himself was required numerous times to rally to these words from the "Ballad of Andrew Barton":

> Fight on…
> I am hurt but I am not slain.
> I'll lay me down and bleed a while,
> Then I'll rise and fight again.

Dennis Raphael
Toronto

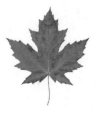

ABOUT CANADA

From health care to agriculture, childcare, globalization, immigration, energy, water and more: the books in this series explore key issues for Canadians. About Canada books provide basic — but critical and passionate — coverage of central aspects of our society. Written in accessible language by experts in their fields, the books are presented in a popular format, at affordable prices.